# Diabetic keratopathy causes vision problems.

Grant M. Taylor

# ACKNOWLEDGEMENTS

First and foremost, I would like to express my deepest gratitude to my mentor, Dr. Jian-Xing Ma, who is truly one of the finest mentors in the world. I feel incredibly fortunate to have him as my mentor and role model. Throughout my Ph.D. journey, Dr. Ma has been a constant source of guidance and support, always available with boundless patience, unparalleled expertise, and a tireless work ethic. Without him, my scientific career would not have been achievable.

I am extremely grateful to the members of my dissertation committee, Dr. Jiyang Cai, Dr. Dimitrios Karamichos, Dr. Michelle Callegan, Dr. Raju Rajala, and Dr. Shaoning Jiang, who have dedicated their time and expertise to guiding me through my graduate studies. Their advice, knowledge, and encouragement have been invaluable to me throughout the entire process of my graduate training. I cannot thank them enough for their dedicated support.

I am deeply thankful to Dr. Gennadiy Moiseyev, Dr. Yusuke Takahashi, and Dr. Rui (Rachel) Cheng for their crucial role in my education. Their guidance, expert advice, and practical assistance were essential to my laboratory work and animal experiments. I am also grateful to all the current and former members of my lab, especially to Dr. Xiang (Eric) Ma, Dr. Wenjing (Lily) Wu, and Mr. Marcus Dehdarani, for their steadfast support and friendship throughout my time in the lab. Their contributions have been invaluable to my academic and personal growth.

I am deeply grateful to Dr. Siribhinya Benyajati and Dr. Hui-Ying Lim, for their constant support and guidance throughout my doctoral education. Their dedication to helping me succeed and their willingness to offer their expertise and advice have been instrumental to my academic growth. I cannot thank them enough for their constant support. I am also grateful to the faculty and staff of the OUHSC Department of Physiology who have assisted me in various ways during my time at the college.

Lastly, I would like to extend my sincerest gratitude to my family, who have provided me with unyielding love and support throughout my journey. I would like to give special recognition to my wife, Li Huang, who has selflessly stood by me and encouraged me to pursue my studies. Her unwavering support has been the foundation of my success and I would not have been able to complete my graduate studies without her. This dissertation is dedicated to my beloved wife, and our two charming children, Aiden and Allison, who are the lights of my life.

# TABLE OF CONTENTS

## LIST OF FIGURES

Figure                                              Page

## ABSTRACT

Diabetes Mellitus is a chronic disease that leads to long-term damage and dysfunction of various organs, such as the eyes, kidneys, nerves, heart, and blood vessels. Diabetic keratopathy is a significant ocular complication of diabetes that leads to persistent corneal epithelial defects and is a major cause of blindness due to its deviation from the normal wound healing process. Despite its significance, the pathogenic mechanism of diabetic keratopathy remains elusive and has received less attention compared to other diabetic complications due to its latent and chronic nature.

The goal of this dissertation is to gain a deeper understanding of the disrupted cornea wound healing process in individuals with diabetes. It is well established that the activation of the canonical Wnt signaling pathway plays a crucial role in regulating cell proliferation, differentiation, and migration. Our studies have revealed that diabetes-induced upregulation of kallistatin potentially contributes to the delayed skin wound healing through inhibition of canonical Wnt signaling. Additionally, our lab has previously shown that Peroxisome Proliferator-Activated Receptor-alpha (PPARα) is down-regulated in diabetic corneas and has neuroprotective effects in diabetic keratopathy. However, the impact of the dysregulation of the Wnt pathway and PPARα signaling on corneal wound healing has not yet been thoroughly studied.

To address the need for a better understanding of the pathogenesis of impaired corneal wound healing in diabetes, this dissertation aims to investigate the pathogenic mechanisms of diabetic keratopathy. The results of my research show that the activation of canonical Wnt signaling is suppressed in the wounded cornea of diabetic mice, which is caused by the upregulated expression of kallistatin and leads to delayed wound healing. Moreover, the study demonstrates that levels of PPARα in the corneal epithelium are significantly reduced in both diabetic patients and animal models, and this reduction correlates with impaired mitochondrial function and delayed corneal wound healing. The identification of the pathogenic mechanism underlying diabetic keratopathy and the development of effective treatments would significantly enhance the quality of life for individuals with diabetes and alleviate the harmful consequences of this serious condition.

CHAPTER I

INTRODUCTION AND LITERATURE REVIEW

CORNEAL STRUCTURE AND FUNCTION

The cornea is a transparent, dome-shaped structure that forms the front surface of the eye (1). It covers the iris, pupil, and anterior chamber. The cornea is responsible for refracting light onto the retina. Besides that, the cornea also serves other important functions, including protecting the inner structures of the eye from physical and chemical damage, maintaining the clarity and transparency of the front of the eye, and helping regulate fluid balance within the eye.

Normal human cornea is avascular. The cornea receives its nutrition primarily from the tear fluid through the outside surface and the aqueous humor through the inside surface. Nutrients are also supplied by the nerve fibers of the cornea (2).

The cornea is composed of five layers: epithelium, Bowman's layer, stroma, Descemet's membrane, and endothelium (Figure 1.1). The corneal epithelium is the outermost layer of the cornea and is composed of 5 – 7 layers of squamous epithelial cells that form a protective barrier against infection and injury. The corneal epithelium plays an important role in maintaining the cornea's transparency. The epithelium is constantly regenerating, and corneal epithelial cells have a lifespan of 7 to 10 days (1). The Bowman's layer (also known as Bowman's membrane) is a thin layer of acellular tissue located between the corneal epithelium and the corneal stroma. It is a crucial part of the cornea's structure, serving as a barrier to protect the stroma from damage. The Bowman's layer is made up of tightly packed Type I and V collagen as well as proteoglycans, which provide its strength and rigidity. It helps maintain the cornea's shape and clarity. The corneal stroma is the middle and thickest layer of the cornea. It is composed of keratocytes and

11

extracellular matrix (ECM) that give the cornea its strength and rigidity (3). The ECM is composed of collagens (Type I, III, V, VI) and glycosaminoglycans (4). The stroma makes up about 80 - 85% of the cornea's thickness, and its transparency is essential for clear vision. The Descemet's membrane (also known as Descemet's layer) is a thin, transparent layer of tissue located between the corneal stroma and the corneal endothelium, next to the inner chamber of the eye. It is composed of Type IV collagen and laminin which are continuously secreted by endothelial cells (1). The corneal endothelium is a single layer of cells located at the innermost part of the cornea, next to the inner chamber of the eye. It contains membrane-bound $Na^+$ $K^+$ ATPase and the intracellular carbonic anhydrase pathway (5), which are essential for regulating the movement of ions and fluid across the endothelial cells (6). These pathways play a critical role in maintaining the fluid balance and transparency of the cornea, as well as regulating the homeostasis of the endothelium. Unlike corneal epithelium, the cells of the endothelium do not regenerate (6).

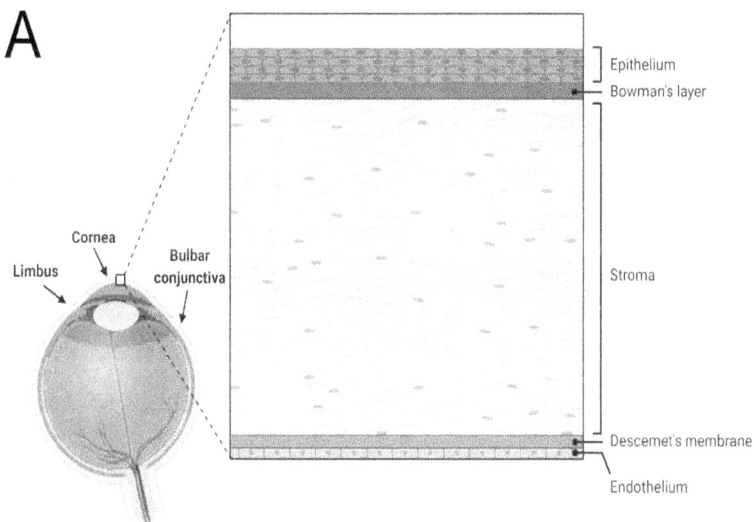


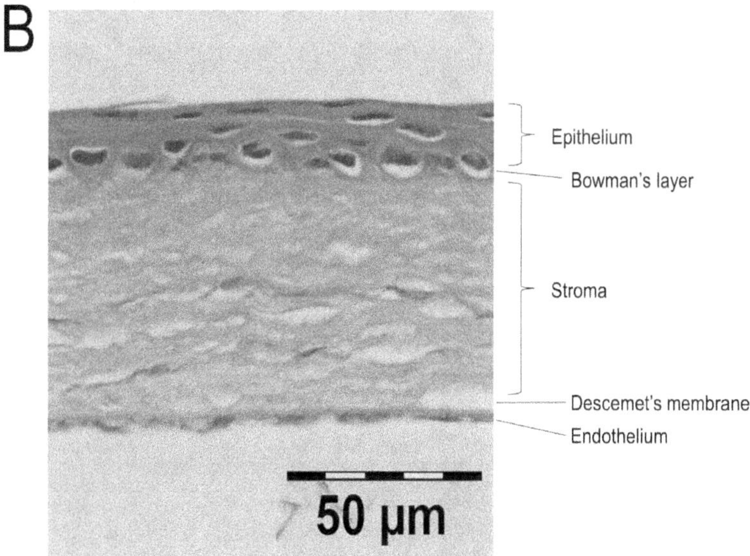


**Figure 1.1 Anatomy of cornea.**
(A) Anatomy of the ocular surface and histology of the human cornea and its various layers. Adapted from Zhang X, Mélik-Parsadaniantz S, Baudouin C, Réaux-Le Goazigo A, Moreau N. Shedding New Light on the Role of Hedgehog Signaling in Corneal Wound Healing. *Int. J. Mol. Sci.* 2022, 23, 3630. (B) Representative H&E staining image of mouse corneal section. Scale bar, 50 µm.

Corneal wound healing is a process by which the eye repairs damage to the cornea. Corneal wound healing typically involves various cellular processes, including proliferation and migration of epithelial cells, interactions between epithelial cells and stromal fibroblasts, and recruitment of various growth factors (7). This process typically occurs in several stages: inflammation, proliferation, maturation, and remodeling (8). After an injury, the eye's immune system responds, and bone marrow-derived cells include monocytes, macrophages, lymphocytes, fibrocytes and other cells enter the area to clean up any debris and help prevent infection (9; 10; 11). Corneal epithelial cells begin to grow and migrate over the wound site to repair the cornea. This process is facilitated by the release of growth factors and signaling molecules that stimulate cell division and migration. Finally, the cornea continues to heal and reorganize, leading to the complete restoration of its transparency and function.

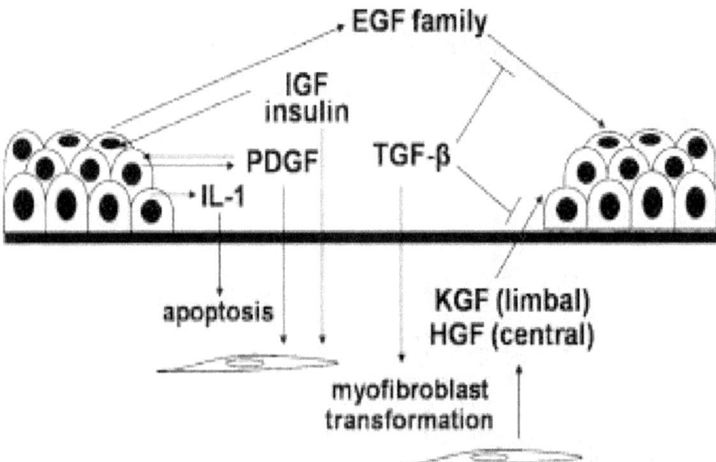


**Figure 1.2 Epithelial wound healing in the cornea involves the release of multiple growth factors and cytokines.**
Keratocytes produce Keratinocyte Growth Factor (KGF) and Hepatocyte Growth Factor (HGF), which influence epithelial behavior. Epithelial secretion of Interleukin-1 (IL-1) and Platelet-Derived Growth Factor (PDGF) modulates stromal response. Epidermal Growth Factor (EGF) family, Insulin-like Growth Factor (IGF), and Transforming Growth Factor-beta (TGF-β) regulate cell transformation and impact wound outcome. The crosstalk among these factors determines the

healing process. Adapted from Yu FS, Yin J, Xu K, Huang J. Growth factors and corneal epithelial wound healing. *Brain Res Bull*. 2010 Feb 15;81(2-3):229-35.

Corneal wound healing is a delicate and complex process that is influenced by various factors, including the cause and extent of the injury, the presence of underlying health conditions, and the individual's overall health and immune system. The treatment for a corneal wound depends on the severity and type of injury. Pain relievers, such as acetaminophen or ibuprofen, can be used to manage pain associated with corneal injury. If there is a risk of infection, topical or oral antibiotics may be prescribed to prevent or treat infection. Artificial tears or ointments may be used to soothe and hydrate the cornea and prevent drying and further injury. In some cases, a protective shield or patch may be placed over the affected eye to prevent further injury and promote healing. In severe cases of corneal injury or disease, corneal wounds may not heal properly and may require medical, such as steroids or topical growth factors, or surgical intervention to promote corneal healing and reduce inflammation (12).

## DIABETIC KERATOPATHY

Diabetes Mellitus is a chronic metabolic disorder characterized by high levels of glucose in the blood (13). The disease is caused by a deficiency of insulin, a hormone produced by the pancreas that regulates blood sugar levels. Diabetes Mellitus is also caused by decreased sensitivity of end organs (such as kidneys, eyes, blood vessels, feet) to insulin action (13). Insulin deficiency can occur due to autoimmune destruction of pancreatic cells, genetic mutations, or lifestyle factors such as obesity, lack of physical activity, and poor diet (13). According to the International Diabetes Federation (IDF), around 537 million people worldwide have diabetes, and this number is expected to rise to 700 million by 2045 (14). The prevalence of diabetes is increasing at an alarming rate, especially in low- and middle-income countries. In 2019, an estimated 4.2 million deaths were attributed to diabetes, making it one of the leading causes of death worldwide (14).

Diabetes Mellitus is associated with long-term damage, dysfunction, and failure of various organs, especially the eyes, kidneys, nerves, heart, and blood vessels (15). Diabetic keratopathy is one of the most blinding diabetic ocular complications and are observed in 45–70% of diabetic patients (7; 16; 17; 18). Diabetic keratopathy can include corneal epithelial defects, decreased corneal sensitivity, corneal nerve alterations, and impaired wound healing. The clinical appearance of diabetic keratopathy can vary depending on the stage and severity of the disease (Figure 1.2). In early stages, the cornea may appear normal or slightly hazy, and there may be no visible signs of inflammation. As the disease progresses, the cornea may become increasingly opaque and develop irregularities, such as epithelial defects, edema, and neovascularization. In severe cases, corneal thinning, scarring, and perforation may occur, leading to permanent vision loss.

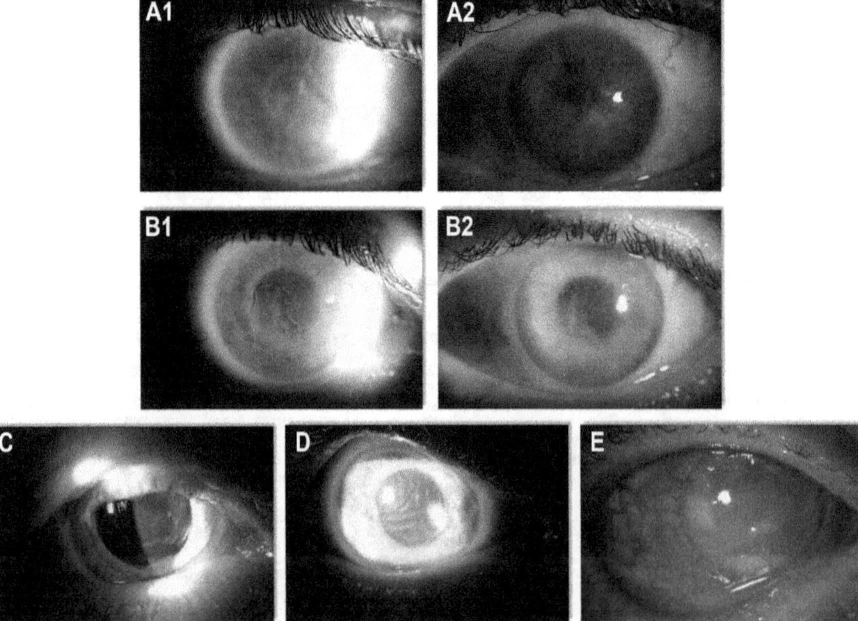


**Figure 1.3 Representative images of common clinical manifestations of diabetic keratopathy.**

(A) Sclerotic scatter illumination slit lamp photograph of the (A1) right and (A2) left eyes highlights areas of central stromal partial light-blocking scarring with adjacent irregular hyperplastic epithelium. Significant superior, nasal, and inferior neovascularization is present. (B) Sclerotic scatter illumination slit lamp photograph of the (B1) right and (B2) left eye demonstrates diffuse stromal edema, Descemet folds, and microcystic edema after cataract surgery. A vertical corneal epithelial defect is also present. (C) Slit lamp photograph of the right eye demonstrates epithelial irregularity and redundant basement membrane in a patient with diabetic keratopathy and epithelial basement membrane disease causing recurrent corneal erosions. (D) Slit lamp photograph of the right eye demonstrates florid stromal folds and edema occupying most of the cornea with limbal sparing. Several bullae are seen superiorly. (E) Slit lamp photograph of the right eye demonstrates 3+ conjunctival injection with significant epithelial defect occupying approximately 60–70% of the cornea with infiltrate. Prominent corneal neovascularization of 360 degrees of the cornea at multiple levels is also present. A 2-mm hypopyon is seen in the anterior chamber. Adapted from Priyadarsini S, Whelchel A, Nicholas S, Sharif R, Riaz K, Karamichos D. Diabetic keratopathy: Insights and challenges. *Surv Ophthalmol.* 2020 Sep-Oct;65(5):513-529.

Although the exact pathogenic mechanisms underlying diabetic keratopathy are not fully understood, several factors have been identified as potential contributors. There are some of the pathogenic mechanisms that may play a role in diabetic keratopathy. Diabetes can lead to corneal epithelial cell dysfunction. Elevated blood glucose levels and oxidative stress can disrupt the normal functioning of the corneal epithelial cells (19; 20), leading to decreased corneal sensitivity, delayed wound healing, and increased susceptibility to infections. Diabetes is associated with peripheral neuropathy, including damage to the nerves supplying the cornea. The corneal nerves play a crucial role in maintaining corneal integrity and sensitivity. The loss of trophic support resulting from corneal neuropathy contributes to damage on the epithelial surface in diabetes (21). Nerve damage can lead to decreased corneal sensation, reduced tear production, and impaired corneal epithelial healing (2). Diabetes can affect the composition of the tear film, which is important for maintaining a healthy ocular surface. Diabetic individuals may experience decreased tear production, changes in tear osmolarity, and altered levels of various tear components, including growth factors and cytokines (22). These changes can contribute to dry eye symptoms, inflammation, and impaired corneal healing. Limbal stem cell dysfunction is another important pathogenic mechanism implicated in diabetic keratopathy. The corneal epithelium is continuously renewed and regenerated by limbal stem cells (LSCs) residing in the basal epithelial layer of the limbus. In individuals with diabetes, studies have observed a significant decrease in the expression of LSC markers within the diabetic limbus (23; 24). Similarly, both type 1 and type 2 diabetic mice have demonstrated a notable reduction in LSC marker expression within the corneal limbus (25; 26). These findings suggest that the loss or dysfunction of resident LSCs may contribute to delayed corneal epithelial wound healing in individuals with diabetic keratopathy. Chronic low-grade inflammation is a hallmark of diabetes. In the context of diabetic keratopathy, increased levels of pro-inflammatory cytokines and chemokines can promote ocular surface inflammation, compromising the integrity of the cornea and exacerbating epithelial cell dysfunction (2).

Diabetic keratopathy can be generally described as a deviation from the normal wound healing mechanism leading to persistent corneal epithelial defects (27; 28). Elevated blood glucose levels, reduced growth factor levels, and altered extracellular matrix composition can all interfere with the regenerative processes necessary for proper corneal repair (27; 28). This impairment can lead to delayed epithelial closure, persistent epithelial defects, and corneal ulcers.

The treatment of diabetic keratopathy depends on the severity of the condition and the underlying cause (27). It is important for people with diabetes to manage their blood sugar levels and undergo regular eye exams to detect diabetic keratopathy and prevent the progression of diabetic keratopathy. Wearing protective eyewear can help prevent further damage to the cornea. Eyedrops and ointments can be used to relieve symptoms and promote corneal healing. In some cases, surgery may be required to remove damaged tissue or repair a corneal ulcer. In severe cases, a corneal transplant may be necessary to restore vision. However, the pathogenic pathways mediating diabetic keratopathy remain uncertain and as such, diabetic keratopathy lacks effective therapy.

## CANONICAL WNT SIGNALING

The canonical Wnt/β-catenin signaling pathway is known to mediate cell proliferation, differentiation and migration (29). Wnt signaling is a tightly regulated pathway comprised of Wnt ligands, frizzled (Fzd) receptors, and co-receptors, including low-density lipoprotein receptor-related protein 5/6 (LRP5/6), an intracellular signaling molecule cascade, and the effector β-catenin (30).

Non-phosphorylated β-catenin plays an essential role in the canonical Wnt pathway (or Wnt/β-catenin pathway). As showed in Figure 1.3, upon binding of Wnt ligands to the Wnt receptor complex, β-catenin becomes unphosphorylated and stabilized, and the unphosphorylated β-catenin is accumulated in the cytosol and then translocated into the nucleus to activate transcription of target genes (31). On the other hand, when Wnt ligands are absent, β-catenin is degraded through the actions of a complex composed of the proteins Axin, adenomatous polyposis coli (APC), glycogen synthase kinase-3 beta (GSK3β), and casein kinase 1 (CK1). This degradation results in the suppression of the Wnt signaling pathway.

Many endogenous proteins have been identified as Wnt inhibitors, such as DKK1, very-low-density lipoprotein receptor (VLDLR), kallistatin, and pigment epithelium-derived factor (PEDF) (31). We also generated a monoclonal antibody specific for the LRP6 E1E2 domains (Mab2F1), which blocks the Wnt/β-catenin signaling at the receptor level (32). Adenovirus expressing a constitutively active mutant of β-catenin (Ad-S37A) in which the phosphorylation site Ser37 in β-catenin was substituted by Ala (S37A) can increase the Wnt signaling (33). Lithium chloride (LiCl) stabilizes β-catenin by inhibiting GSK-3β and is commonly used to activate canonical Wnt signaling intracellularly (34; 35; 36). Our previous study has also shown that VLDLR inhibits Wnt signaling by dimerizing with LRP6 through its extracellular domain (VLN), and VLDLR ablation results in Wnt signaling overactivation (37; 38; 39).

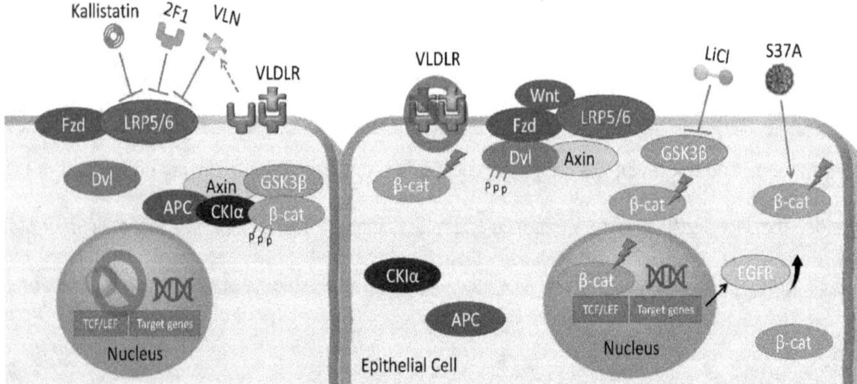


**Figure 1.4 The canonical Wnt signaling.**
Kallistatin protein, an LRP6-blocking antibody (2F1), or soluble VLDLR ectodomain (VLN) inhibit the Wnt/β-catenin signaling. In contrast, lithium chloride (LiCl) or the constitutively active mutant of β-catenin (S37A) activates the Wnt/β-catenin signaling. Ablation of VLDLR also results in the overactivation of Wnt signaling pathway. APC: adenomatous polyposis coli; CKIα: casein kinase Iα; Dvl: Dishevelled; EGFR: epidermal growth factor receptor; Fzd: frizzled receptor; GSK-3β: glycogen synthase kinase 3 beta; LRP5/6: low-density lipoprotein receptor-related protein 5 or 6; TCF/LEF: T-cell factor/lymphoid enhancer factor.

The role of Wnt signaling in different tissues and organs can vary, and its activation can have different effects depending on the context. In the retina and kidney, excessive Wnt activation has been associated with the pathogenesis of several diseases in the retina and kidney (31; 32; 40; 41; 42; 43).

For example, in diabetic retinopathy, Wnt signaling has been shown to promote inflammation and vascular dysfunction, which are key features of the disease (31; 40; 41). Studies have shown that levels of total β-catenin are elevated in retinal sections of patients with non-proliferative diabetic retinopathy compared to those from non-diabetic controls (44). In animal models of diabetic retinopathy, including Akita mice and streptozotocin-induced diabetic rats, β-catenin levels were up-regulated, along with the expression of Wnt co-receptor LRP5/6 (44). Furthermore, studies have found that vitreous samples from patients with proliferative diabetic retinopathy have higher levels of LRP6 compared to non-diabetic controls, and elevated LRP6 levels are correlated with the levels of vascular endothelial growth factor (VEGF) in the vitreous

(45). These findings suggest that Wnt signaling, through its interaction with VEGF, may play a role in the development of proliferative diabetic retinopathy. In humans, serum levels of DKK-1, a Wnt signaling inhibitor, are lower in patients with diabetic retinopathy compared with those from non-diabetic patients or diabetic patients without diabetic retinopathy, further supporting the importance of the Wnt signaling pathway in diabetic retinopathy (46). In addition, studies have shown that pharmacological inhibition of Wnt signaling can attenuate retinal vascular leakage in animal models of diabetic retinopathy. For example, DKK-1 reduced retinal inflammation, ameliorated vascular leakage, and decreased neovascularization in STZ-induced diabetic rats (44). DKK-1 inhibited proliferation and migration of human retinal pigment epithelial (RPE) cells, and the expression of β-catenin and cyclin D1 is decreased in DKK-1 over-expressed RPE cells (47). A monoclonal antibody blocking the Wnt pathway was found to have therapeutic potential in reducing retinal vascular leakage in a mouse model of diabetic retinopathy (32). Another study investigated the potential benefits of Wnt inhibitory factor 1 (WIF1), which can block the Wnt signaling pathway, in treating diabetic retinopathy. The authors found that treatment with WIF1 improved mitochondrial function and reduced inflammation and oxidative stress in the retinas of diabetic mice, potentially through the AMPK/mTOR pathway (48).

Similarly, in renal fibrosis, Wnt signaling has been shown to play a key role in the activation of fibroblasts and the deposition of extracellular matrix proteins in the kidney. Studies have shown that the activation of Wnt signaling is increased in the kidneys of animal models of renal fibrosis and patients with chronic kidney disease, and that pharmacological inhibition of Wnt signaling can attenuate renal fibrosis and improve renal function (43; 49). Moreover, Wnt signaling has been shown to regulate the expression of pro-fibrotic factors and matrix metalloproteinases in renal cells, suggesting that it can contribute to the activation of fibrotic pathways and the deposition of extracellular matrix proteins in the kidney (50; 51).

On the other hand, in skin, Wnt signaling has been shown to promote keratinocyte proliferation and differentiation, which are essential processes for wound healing and skin repair

(52; 53; 54; 55). Specifically, McBride et al. found that impaired Wnt signaling due to elevated levels of an antiangiogenic SERPIN in patients with diabetic microvascular complications leads to impaired wound healing (52). Shi et al. demonstrated that Wnt and Notch signaling pathways are involved in skin wound healing by targeting c-Myc and Hes1 separately (54). Choi et al. reviewed different approaches for regenerative healing of cutaneous wounds, with an emphasis on strategies that activate the Wnt/beta-Catenin pathway (53). And Widelitz provided an overview of the role of Wnt signaling in skin organogenesis and development, which is closely linked to skin wound healing and regeneration (55). Overall, the evidence suggests that Wnt signaling is a critical pathway in promoting keratinocyte proliferation and differentiation, and that its activation may be a promising therapeutic target for promoting skin wound healing and skin repair.

**Wnt Signaling in Cornea**

Several studies have investigated the role of Wnt signaling in the corneal epithelium and its impact on various cellular processes. In 2011, it was observed that Wnt signaling is present in the ocular surface epithelium and plays a crucial role in regulating the proliferation of limbal stem cells (56). A study in 2014 highlighted the importance of Wnt7A in determining cell fate and promoting differentiation of both limbal stem cells and cornea epithelial cells(57). Subsequent research conducted in 2019 demonstrated that corneal keratocyte-derived Wnt/$\beta$-catenin signaling is essential for corneal epithelial maturation during ocular surface development (58). Additionally, it was found that Wnt signaling is required for the maintenance of human limbal stem/progenitor cells in vitro (59; 60). Furthermore, insulin was found to enhance corneal nerve repair and wound healing in type 1 diabetic mice by enhancing Wnt/$\beta$-Catenin signaling (61).

Despite its importance, the specific role of Wnt/$\beta$-catenin signaling in the process of corneal wound repair is not fully understood.

Peroxisome Proliferator-Activated Receptor (PPAR) is a group of transcription factors that belong to the nuclear receptor superfamily (62). There are three main subtypes of PPAR: PPARα, PPARδ, and PPARγ (62; 63). PPARα is primarily expressed in the liver and plays a role in regulating lipid metabolism, while PPARδ is found in various tissues, including muscle and fat, and is involved in regulating energy metabolism. PPARγ is expressed in adipose tissue and the gut and plays a key role in insulin sensitivity and glucose metabolism (63).

PPARα is primarily expressed in tissues with high rates of fatty acid oxidation, such as the liver, heart, and skeletal muscle (64). Upon activation, PPARα heterodimerizes with the Retinoid X Receptor (RXR) and binds to PPAR Response Elements (PPREs) in the promoter regions of target genes including PPARα itself and those involved in many processes such as energy metabolism, oxidative stress, inflammation, circadian rhythm, immune response, mitochondrial genesis and cell differentiation (65; 66; 67; 68; 69; 70; 71).

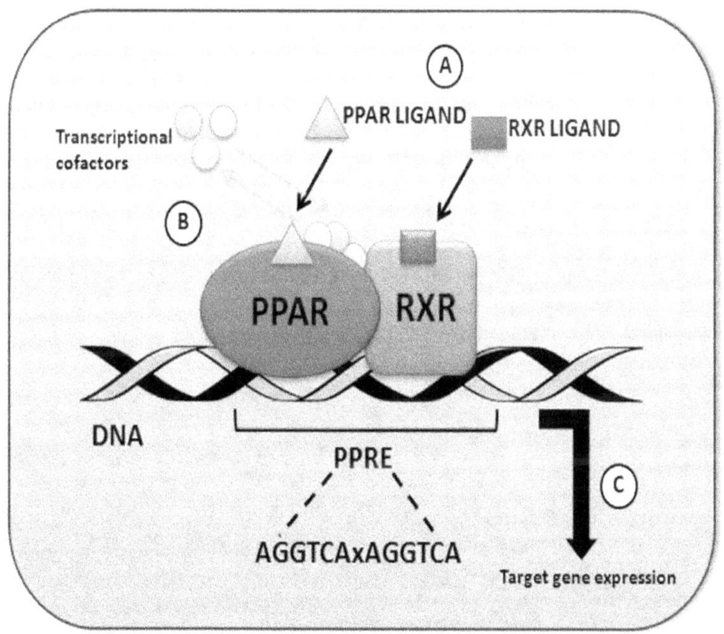

**Figure 1.5 PPAR transcriptional activation in the cell nucleus.**
(A) Binding of PPAR/RXR ligands; (B) Changes in the associated transcriptional cofactors; (C) Activation of the transcriptional complex. Adapted from Rigano D, Sirignano C, Taglialatela-Scafati O. The potential of natural products for targeting PPARα. *Acta Pharm Sin B*. 2017 Jul;7(4):427-438.

PPARα$^{-/-}$ mice were first generated by Dr. Frank Gonzalez using homologous recombination technology and the details of this study were published in the journal Molecular and Cellular Biology in 1995 (72). They found that PPARα$^{-/-}$ mice had abnormal lipid metabolism in the liver, characterized by decreased fatty acid oxidation and increased lipid accumulation. They also showed that PPARα$^{-/-}$ mice were unable to respond to the lipid-lowering effects of fibrates, a class of drugs that activate PPARα.

Two independent, prospective clinical studies reported robust therapeutic effects of PPARα agonist fenofibrate on diabetic retinopathy in type 2 diabetic patients (73). Our previous study has shown that diabetes-induced down-regulation of PPARα in the retina plays a key pathogenic role in retinal oxidative stress and inflammation in diabetic retinopathy (74). Recently, we demonstrated that PPARα protein levels are decreased in the corneal epithelium from both type 1 and type 2 diabetic donors compared to non-diabetic human donors (75). PPARα$^{-/-}$ mice showed declined corneal nerve densities and increased epithelial lesion in the central cornea (75). It has been reported that PPARα agonist accelerated corneal epithelial healing after alkali injury (76). These observations suggested that PPARα has a role in maintenance of corneal integrity. However, the physiological function of PPARα in the cornea, especially in the regulation of mitochondria function, has not been previously investigated.

# MITOCHONDRIAL DYSFUNCTION IN DIABETES

Mitochondria are complex, dynamic organelles found in the cytoplasm of eukaryotic cells that are is referred to as the "powerhouses" of the cell (77). Mitochondria play a central role in cellular metabolism and energy production by generating the majority of a cell's supply of ATP through the process of oxidative phosphorylation (77). In addition to energy production, mitochondria are involved in a number of other cellular processes, including calcium regulation, apoptosis, and oxidative stress response (77; 78; 79). Mitochondria play a crucial role in regulating intracellular calcium levels, which is important for maintaining normal cellular function. Mitochondria are also involved in the regulation of programmed cell death, or apoptosis, which is a normal physiological process that helps to eliminate damaged or abnormal cells.

Mitochondrial dysfunction has been implicated in a wide range of diseases, including cardiovascular disease, diabetes, and neurodegenerative disorders, as well as in aging and age-related diseases (79; 80). Neurodegenerative disorders such as Parkinson's disease, Alzheimer's disease, and Huntington's disease are characterized by progressive loss of brain function and have been linked to mitochondrial dysfunction (81). Mitochondrial dysfunction has been implicated in the development of cardiovascular disease, including heart attacks and stroke (82). Mitochondrial dysfunction has been implicated in the development of insulin resistance and the associated complications of diabetes. Specifically, mitochondrial dysfunction can affect the cells' ability to process glucose and other fuels. In addition, mitochondrial dysfunction can also contribute to oxidative stress and inflammation, which are hallmarks of diabetic complications (83). These processes can cause further damage to the cells and organs affected by diabetes, exacerbating the symptoms and progression of the disease.

Previous studies have indicated a decline in mitochondrial function within corneal cells in individuals with diabetes. Mussi et al. demonstrated that high glucose culture adversely affects mitochondrial function in human telomerase-immortalized corneal epithelial cells (84). Aldrich et al. reported impaired mitochondrial function in corneal endothelial cells from advanced diabetic donors, as assessed by extracellular flux analysis (85). Qu et al. found that the mitochondrial function of the lacrimal gland was more severely compromised in diabetic mice, leading to reduced tear secretion (86). Exposure to low-intensity blue light emitted from computer screens has been found to reduce the proliferation rate of corneal epithelial (HCE-2) cells and induce cell death in a dose-dependent manner, involving mitochondrial dysfunction (87). Insulin has been shown to selectively regulate PTEN-induced kinase 1 (PINK-1)-mediated mitophagy and mitochondrial accumulation of insulin receptor (INSR) in human telomerized corneal epithelial (hTCEpi) cell line (88). Additionally, epidermal growth factor (EGF) has been found to promote damage repair by inducing mitochondrial autophagy and alleviating mitochondrial damage in human corneal epithelial cells (89). Furthermore, healthy mesenchymal stem cells (MSCs) have been shown to donate mitochondria to the cornea and enhance corneal wound healing in a rabbit model (90).

However, the direct contribution of mitochondrial function to the corneal epithelial wound repair process remains incompletely understood. Therefore, further investigation is needed to elucidate the underlying mechanisms of the intricate relationship between diabetic keratopathy and mitochondrial dysfunction. Such research holds promise for the development of novel therapeutic strategies.

## SUMMARY

The focus of this dissertation is to gain a deeper insight into the impaired corneal wound healing process in diabetic keratopathy. Previous research has indicated that diabetes has been linked to an upregulation of kallistatin, which potentially contributes to delayed skin wound healing through inhibition of the Wnt/β-catenin signaling pathway. Furthermore, our studies have shown that the PPARα pathway is downregulated in diabetic corneas and has neuroprotective effects. Mitochondrial dysfunction has been identified as a common mechanism underlying various diabetic complications and could also play a role in the delayed wound healing process. In order to shed light on the pathogenesis of impaired corneal wound healing in diabetes, this dissertation aims to examine the impact of the dysregulation of the Wnt/β-catenin signaling pathway and the PPARα pathway on corneal mitochondria function as well as wound healing. This dissertation revealed that diabetic corneas in humans, rats, and mice exhibited elevated levels of kallistatin, which hindered the activation of canonical Wnt signaling and led to delayed wound healing. Transgenic expression of kallistatin exacerbated this delay. Manipulation of Wnt signaling using inhibitors or activators influenced the rate of corneal wound healing. Additionally, restoring PPARα expression in the corneal epithelium improved mitochondrial function and enhanced wound healing, highlighting the significance of PPARα downregulation in contributing to impaired wound healing in diabetic corneas. By examining the role of mitochondrial dysfunction, Wnt/β-catenin signaling, and PPARα signaling in corneal wound healing, this dissertation contributes to a better understanding of the pathogenesis of impaired corneal wound healing in diabetic keratopathy.

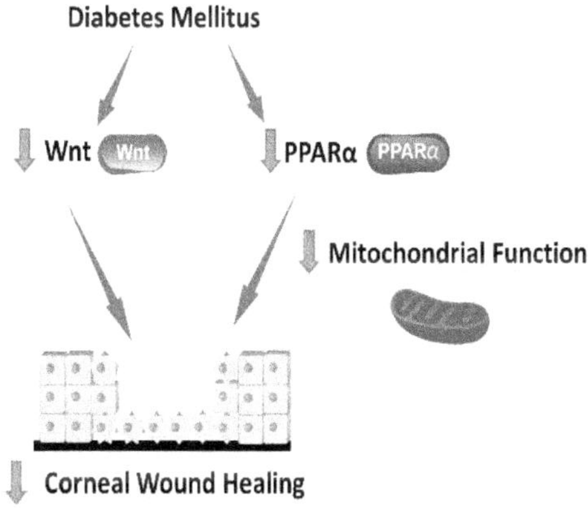


**Figure 1.6 Proposed mechanisms for diabetic keratopathy.**
Decreased Wnt signaling together with PPARα levels in the cornea may account for the pathogenesis of diabetic keratopathy in part.

**CHAPTER II**

**PATHOGENIC ROLE OF DIABETES-INDUCED OVEREXPRESSION OF KALLISTATIN**

**IN CORNEAL WOUND HEALING DEFICIENCY**

**THROUGH INHIBITION OF CANONICAL WNT SIGNALING**

The following chapter is adapted from the published manuscript entitled "Pathogenic Role of Diabetes-induced Overexpression of Kallistatin in Corneal Wound Healing Deficiency through Inhibition of Canonical Wnt Signaling" in the *Diabetes* Journal. Wentao Liang conducted experiments in Figures 2.1 to 2.8. The data in Figures 2.1A-B, 2.2, 2.3, 2.4F-H, 2.5D-E were generated by Li Huang and the data were analyzed by Wentao Liang. Xiang Ma, Lijie Dong, and Rui Cheng provided the experimental animals. Marcus Dehdarani generated the kallistatin protein and Mab2F1 antibody used in this study. Wentao Liang and Li Huang wrote the manuscript. Dimitrios Karamichos and Jian-Xing Ma designed the research, analyzed data, wrote, and edited the manuscript. Citation: "Liang W, Huang L, Ma X, Dong L, Cheng R, Dehdarani M, Karamichos D, Ma JX. Pathogenic Role of Diabetes-Induced Overexpression of Kallistatin in Corneal Wound Healing Deficiency Through Inhibition of Canonical Wnt Signaling. *Diabetes*. 2022 Apr 1;71(4):747-761. doi: 10.2337/db21-0740. PMID: 35044447; PMCID: PMC8965664." The electronic version: https://www.ncbi.nlm.nih.gov/pmc/articles/PMC8965664.

**ABSTRACT**

It was reported previously that circulation levels of kallistatin, an endogenous Wnt signaling inhibitor, are increased in diabetic patients. The present study was to determine the role of kallistatin in delayed wound healing in diabetic cornea. Immunostaining and Western blot analysis showed kallistatin levels were upregulated in diabetic human and rodent corneas. In murine corneal wound healing models, the canonical Wnt signaling was activated in non-diabetic cornea and suppressed in diabetic cornea, correlating with delayed wound healing. Transgenic expression of kallistatin suppressed the activation of Wnt signaling in the cornea and delayed wound healing. Local inhibition of Wnt signaling in the cornea by kallistatin, an LRP6-blocking antibody, or the soluble VLDLR ectodomain (an endogenous Wnt signaling inhibitor) delayed wound healing. In contrast, ablation of VLDLR resulted in overactivation of Wnt/$\beta$-catenin signaling and accelerated corneal wound healing. Activation of Wnt signaling in the cornea accelerated wound healing. Activation of Wnt signaling promoted human corneal epithelial cell migration and proliferation, which was attenuated by kallistatin. Our findings suggested that diabetes-induced overexpression of kallistatin contributes to delayed corneal wound healing by inhibiting the canonical Wnt signaling. Thus, kallistatin and Wnt/$\beta$-catenin signaling in the cornea could be potential therapeutic targets for diabetic corneal complications.

**INTRODUCTION**

Diabetes Mellitus (DM) is a metabolic disorder of complex etiology characterized by chronic hyperglycemia with disturbed metabolism of carbohydrate, fat, and protein resulting from defects in insulin secretion, insulin action, or both (13). DM is associated with long-term damage, dysfunction, and failure of various organs, especially the eye, kidney, nerve, heart, and blood vessel (13). A smooth and continuous surface of the cornea is essential for normal vision. However, compared to other diabetic complications, diabetic keratopathy (DK), one of the blinding diabetic ocular complications, receives less attention. Diabetes results in reduced corneal epithelial cell density and sub-basal nerve plexus alterations (91; 92; 93; 94). The effect and underline mechanism of altered metabolism in diabetic patients on ocular surface wound healing remains unclear. Previous studies have reported that elevated serum levels of tumor necrosis factor-α (TNF-α), interleukin (IL)-6 and IL-8 in patients with diabetes could contribute to the diabetic corneal complication (94; 95). On the other hand, hyperglycemia changed the expression of cytokines in the cornea, such as reduced levels of Insulin Growth Factor-1 (IGF-1), Transforming Growth Factor Beta 3 (TGFβ3), Epidermal Growth Factor Receptor (EGFR), and Ciliary Neurotrophic Factor (CNTF), which may contribute to the delayed cornea wound healing in diabetic condition (96; 97). However, the pathogenic pathways mediating DK remain uncertain.

The Wnt/β-catenin signaling pathway is known to mediate cell proliferation, differentiation and migration (29). Wnt signaling is a tightly regulated pathway comprised of Wnt ligands, frizzled (Fzd) receptors, and co-receptors, including low-density lipoprotein receptor-related protein 5/6 (LRP5/6), an intracellular signaling molecule cascade and the effector β-catenin (30). Non-phosphorylated β-catenin plays an essential role in the canonical Wnt pathway (or Wnt/β-catenin pathway). Upon binding of Wnt ligands to the Wnt receptor complex, β-catenin becomes unphosphorylated, and the unphosphorylated β-catenin is accumulated in the cytosol and then translocated into the nucleus to activate transcription of target genes (31).

Wnt signaling dysregulation in diabetes conditions is tissue specific. For example, we found that Wnt signaling is over-activated in the retina from diabetic patients or diabetic animal models (31; 32; 42). Furthermore, aberrant activation of canonical Wnt signaling leads to retinal inflammation and neovascularization (31; 32; 40; 41; 42). However, diabetes suppressed Wnt signaling in the skin, contributing to delayed skin wound healing (52). Recently, a study suggested that Wnt signaling may mediate the beneficial effect of insulin on corneal wound healing (61). However, the mechanism for the dysregulation of Wnt signaling in the cornea in diabetes is unclear.

Many endogenous proteins have been identified as Wnt inhibitors, such as DKK1, very-low-density lipoprotein receptor (VLDLR), kallistatin, and pigment epithelium-derived factor (PEDF) (31). We also generated a monoclonal antibody specific for the LRP6 E1E2 domains (Mab2F1), which blocks the Wnt/$\beta$-catenin signaling at the receptor level (32). Our previous study has shown that VLDLR inhibits Wnt signaling by dimerizing with LRP6 through its extracellular domain (VLN), and VLDLR ablation results in Wnt signaling overactivation (37; 38; 39). However, the impacts of kallistatin, Mab2F1 and VLDLR on the canonical Wnt pathway activity in diabetic cornea and their roles in corneal wound healing remains elusive.

Kallistatin is a serine proteinase inhibitor (98; 99). We reported previously that kallistatin protein functions as an endogenous antagonist of LRP6 and inhibitor of Wnt signaling in the retina (100). Decreased kallistatin levels were found in the vitreous of diabetic patients and the retina of diabetic animal models (101). However, circulating kallistatin levels are elevated in both type 1 and type 2 diabetic patients with complications (102). The elevated kallistatin level is responsible, at least in part, for the delayed skin wound healing in diabetes through inhibition of Wnt signaling (52). However, the impact of kallistatin on diabetic corneas has not been well studied.

In the present study, we first quantified the expression level of kallistatin in the diabetic human cornea. We hypothesized that elevated kallistatin levels suppressed Wnt/$\beta$-catenin signaling in diabetic corneas, leading to delayed corneal wound healing. To investigate the pathogenic role of Wnt signaling in the context of corneal wound healing, we measured Wnt signaling activities in the corneas of type 1 diabetic mouse models and corneal wound healing rate. To further investigate the role of kallistatin and Wnt signaling in corneal wound healing, we modulated Wnt/β-catenin activities using genetic and pharmacological approaches and evaluated their impacts on the corneal wound healing rate. We also evaluated the roles of kallistatin and Wnt signaling in the proliferation and migration of human corneal epithelial cells (HCEC) *in vitro*.

## RESEARCH DESIGN AND METHODS

### Ethical approval and informed consent

The study adhered to the tenets of the Declaration of Helsinki and was performed with the Institutional Review Board (IRB) approval from the University of Oklahoma Health Sciences Center (protocol #3450). Donor eyes from patients with diabetes and age-matched patients without diabetes were obtained from Lions Gift of Sight eye bank (Saint Paul, MN). All methods were performed in accordance with federal and institutional guidelines and all human samples were de-identified prior to analysis. Clinical data for the non-diabetic (NDM) and diabetic (DM) donors are as followed. NDM: 3 females and 3 males, all Caucasian, and the average age was 77.8 years. Cause of death included COPD, cardiac arrest, sepsis, Alzheimer's disease, intracranial bleeding (ICB) and intracerebral hemorrhage (ICH). DM: 1 female and 5 males whose average age was 75 years, all Caucasian. All of them had diabetes for more than 10 years. Cause of death included pancreatic cancer, sepsis, dementia, gastroesophageal junction adenocarcinoma and pneumonia.

### Animals

Male Brown Norway (BN) rats (8–10 week-old; Charles River, Wilmington, MA), kallistatin transgenic (KS-Tg) mice in the C57/BL/6J background overexpressing human kallistatin (12-20 week-old, generated as described previously (100)), wild-type (WT) C57BL/6J mice, Akita (*Ins2^{akita}*) mice (16-20 week-old), *db/db* (BKS.Cg- *Lepr^{db}*/J) mice (16-20 week-old), *Vldlr^{-/-}* mice (12-20 week-old) and Axin2-lacZ reporter mice (12-20 week-old; Jackson Laboratories, Bar Harbor, ME) were used. All experiments were performed following the guidelines of the ARVO Statement for the Use of Animals in Ophthalmic and Vision Research and approved by the Institutional Animal Care and Use Committee of the University of Oklahoma Health Sciences Center. In all procedures, animals were anesthetized with i.p. injection of 50 mg/kg ketamine hydrochloride mixed with 5 mg/kg xylazine (Vedco, St. Joseph, MO).

## Induction of diabetes by streptozotocin (STZ) injection

Diabetes was induced in mice and rats at 8-week of age as described previously (103; 104). Briefly, mice received 5 daily intraperitoneal injections of freshly prepared STZ (Sigma-Aldrich Corp.; 55 mg/kg in 10 mM of citrate buffer, pH 4.5), while BN rats received a single intraperitoneal injection of STZ following overnight fasting. Age-matched mice and rats that received citrate buffer injection alone were used for non-diabetic controls. Animals with blood glucose levels higher than 350 mg/dL were considered diabetic.

## Corneal epithelial debridement wound

The corneal wound was induced following a documented protocol (105). After anesthesia, the central corneal epithelial layer was removed with an Algerbrush II Corneal Rust Ring Remover (Alloy Medical, San Mateo, CA) with a diameter of 2-mm in mice and 4-mm in rats. The abraded region was labeled with 0.1% sodium fluorescein and photographed daily with Micron IV (Phoenix Technology Group, Pleasanton, CA). The wound area was quantified with Image J software (National Institutes of Health, Bethesda, MD).

## Immunohistochemistry of human eyes

Human donor eyes dissected within 12 hr postmortem were immediately preserved in Davidson's fixation solution for 24 hr and then transferred to 10% buffered formalin for storage and paraffin section. Following the antigen retrieval with ethylenediaminetetraacetic acid (EDTA) buffer (1 mM EDTA, 0.05% Tween 20, pH 8.0) in steam bath and blocking, the sections were incubated with an anti-human kallistatin antibody (R&D #AF1669) overnight. After washes with phosphate-buffered saline (PBS), the slides were incubated with A488 labeled donkey anti-goat IgG (Jackson ImmunoResearch #705-545-003). The slides were mounted with Vectashield mounting buffer containing DAPI (Vector Laboratories #H-1200) and then photographed under a fluorescence microscope (Observer Z1, Pleasanton, CA).

**Immunohistochemistry of rat and mouse corneas**

Anti-rat kallistatin antibody expressed in mouse hybridoma cell was generated through a contracted service at ProteinTech company (Rosemont, IL). The rat and mouse eyeballs were fixed in Davidson's fixation solution for 48 h for the paraffin section. Following the antigen retrieval with sodium citrate buffer (10 mM sodium citrate, 0.05% Tween 20, pH 6.0) in steam bath and blocking, the sections were incubated with anti-rat kallistatin antibody or anti-non-phosphorylated β-catenin antibody (Cell Signaling #8814) overnight. After washed with PBS, the slides were incubated with A488 labeled goat anti-mouse IgG (Jackson ImmunoResearch #115-545-003) or A488 labeled goat anti-rabbit IgG (Jackson ImmunoResearch #111-545-003). The slides were mounted with Vectashield mounting buffer containing DAPI (Vector Laboratories #H-1200) and photographed under a Zeiss Microscope (Observer Z1, Pleasanton, CA).

**X-gal staining**

The X-Gal staining was performed following the instruction of the manufacturer. Briefly, the corneas were fixed in 4% paraformaldehyde in 1× PBS pH 7.4 (PFA/PBS) for 30 min at 4°C , and then stained with the X-gal staining solution (5 mM potassium ferricyanide, 5 mM potassium ferrocyanide, 2 mM $MgCl_2$, 0.02% NP-40, 0.01% sodium deoxycholate, 0.4 mg/ml X-gal in PBS) overnight (106; 107). Corneas were flat-mounted with mounting media (Immu-Mount; Thermo Fisher Scientific, Inc. Kalamazoo, MI), and photographed under an Olympus Microscope (BX43F; Olympus, Tokyo, Japan).

## Human corneal epithelial cell (HCEC) viability assay

HCEC (ATCC #PCS700010) were cultured in Corneal Epithelial Cell Basal Medium (ATCC #PCS700030) in a 24-well plate. After incubation with 20% L cell-conditioned medium (LCM) or Wnt3a conditioned medium (WCM) and different concentrations of human kallistatin protein. The cell suspension was stained with trypan blue (ThermoFisher). Viable cells were counted using Cellometer Auto T4 Bright Field Cell Counter (Nexcelom, Lawrence, MA).

## Cell migration assay

HCEC were treated with WCM and various concentrations of kallistatin after 100% confluence. *In vitro* "wound" was created by a straight-line scratch across the monolayer using a 200 µL pipette tip as described previously (108). Then 6 images of each scratch were taken by Cytation 1 Cell Imaging Multi-Mode Reader (BioTek; Winooski, VT) at different time points. The acellular area was measured using the Image J Program.

## Western blot analysis

Western blot analysis was performed as described previously (109). Anti-human kallistatin monoclonal antibodies were gifts from Drs. L. Chao and J. Chao (98; 99). GAPDH (abcam #ab9485), rabbit anti-kallistatin antibody (abcam #ab187656), anti-non-phosphorylated β-catenin antibody (Cell Signaling #8814), anti-EGFR antibody (abcam #ab52894) and mouse anti-β-actin antibody (Sigma-Aldrich #A5441) were used as primary antibodies at 1:1000 dilution. Horseradish peroxidase-labeled secondary antibodies (1:2000 dilution, Santa Cruz Biotechnology) were used for immunoblotting. Densitometry was performed using ImageJ software and normalized by β-actin levels.

## Statistical analysis

All statistical analyses were carried out using GraphPad Prism 9 (GraphPad Software, Inc., Boston, MA). Data were expressed as mean ± SEM. The paired Student's *t*-test was applied to compare differences between two groups. ANOVA was used to compare three or more groups.

**Upregulated expression of kallistatin in diabetic human, rat and murine corneas**

To study whether kallistatin is expressed in the cornea and its expression is altered in diabetes, we performed immunostaining of kallistatin in diabetic human corneas. The result showed that kallistatin levels were upregulated in the cornea epithelium from diabetic human donors, compared with those in non-diabetic subjects (Figure 2.1A). Similarly, kallistatin levels were increased in the cornea epithelial layer of STZ-induced diabetic rats (3 months of diabetes), compared with that in the non-diabetic controls (Figure 2.1B). We also performed Western blot analysis of kallistatin in tissue lysate from diabetic human corneas. The result showed that there was a trend of upregulated kallistatin levels in the corneas from human donors with diabetes, compared with those in the non-diabetic subjects (Figure 2.1C). As shown by Western blot analysis, the kallistatin level was upregulated in the corneas of type 1 diabetes mouse models (Akita mice and STZ-induced diabetic mice) and type 2 diabetes mouse model (*db/db* mice), compared with those in the respective non-diabetic controls (Figure 2.1D-F).

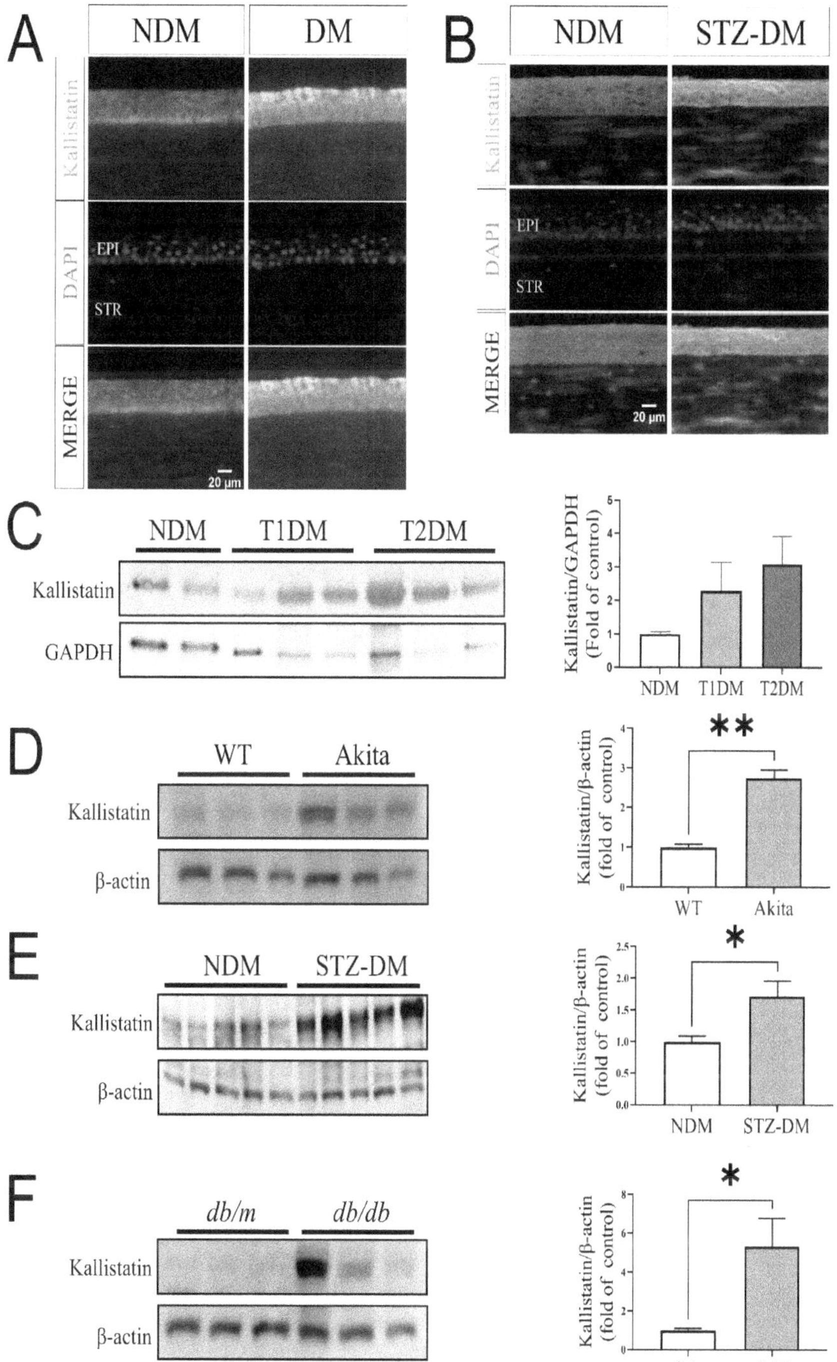



Figure 2.1 Kallistatin protein levels in non-diabetic and diabetic corneas.

(A) Representative immunostaining images of kallistatin (green) and DAPI (blue) in the corneas from non-diabetic (NDM) and diabetic (DM) donors (n=6). EPI: epithelium. STR: stroma. (B) Representative immunostaining images of kallistatin (green) and DAPI (blue) in the corneas from STZ-induced diabetic rats (STZ, 3 months of diabetes) and NDM controls (n=3). (C) Representative images of Western blotting of kallistatin in the corneas were collected from non-diabetic (NDM), type 1 diabetic (T1DM), and type 2 diabetic (T2DM) donors. Densitometry analysis of kallistatin in the cornea and normalized by GAPDH as a loading control (mean ± SEM). NDM (n=2), T1DM (n=3), and T2DM (n=3). (D, E, F) Representative Western blots for kallistatin and densitometry quantification in the corneas from Akita mice (n=3), STZ-induced DM mice (n=5), and *db/db* mice (n=3), and their respective NDM controls. All values are mean ± SEM. *P<0.05, **P<0.01.

## Increased Wnt/β-catenin signaling activities in the corneas with wound healing

To examine the activation of the Wnt/β-catenin pathway in the corneal wound healing process, we measured non-phosphorylated β-catenin in wounded corneas in WT mice. As shown in Figure 2.2A, elevated levels of non-phosphorylated β-catenin were detected in the wounded corneas compared with that in the unwounded corneas, suggesting that Wnt signaling was activated in the cornea in response to wounding. A canonical Wnt reporter mouse line, the Axin2-lacZ mouse line, was used to confirm the activation of corneal Wnt signaling during wound healing (107). At 48 hr after epithelial debridement, the corneas were stained with X-gal. The wounded corneas showed more intense X-gal staining compared with unwounded corneas (Figure 2.2B). These data indicated that the Wnt pathway is activated during the epithelial wound healing process.

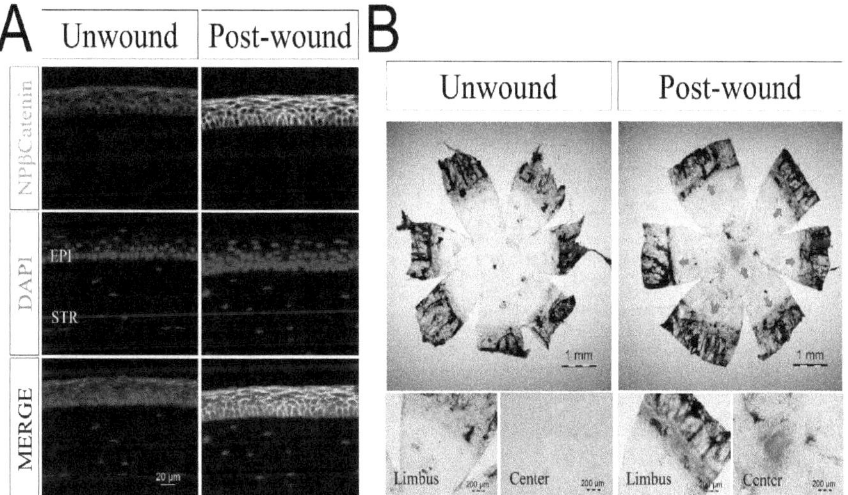


**Figure 2.2 Increased Wnt/β-catenin signaling activities in the corneas with wound healing.** (A) Representative immunostaining images of non-phosphorylated β-catenin (NP-β-catenin, green) and DAPI (blue) in corneal sections of 5-month-old C57BL/6J mice with corneal wound and age-matched unwound controls (n=5). EPI: epithelium. STR: stroma. (B) Representative images of X-gal staining (blue) of flat-mounted corneas from Axin2-LacZ mice with and without wound (n=5).

**Diabetic corneas showed attenuated Wnt/β-catenin signaling activation and delayed wound healing**

At 12 weeks after the onset of STZ-induced diabetes, diabetic C57BL/6J mice were subjected to corneal wound healing. On both day 2 and day 3 post wounding, the epithelial depletion areas were significantly larger in diabetic mice than those of age-matched non-diabetic mice (Figure 2.3A and 2.3B). Similarly, the delayed epithelial wound closure was also observed in Akita mice, a genetic type 1 diabetic model (Figure 2.3C) and STZ-induced diabetic rats (Figure 2.3D). These findings demonstrated delayed corneal epithelial wound healing in diabetic animals.

As shown by immunostaining, the non-phosphorylated β-catenin level was declined in the wounded corneal epithelium of Akita mice or STZ-induced diabetic mice, compared with that in the respective non-diabetic controls (Figure 2.3E and 2.3F).

Taken together, these data revealed that the activation of Wnt/β-catenin signaling is suppressed in diabetic corneas during wound healing.

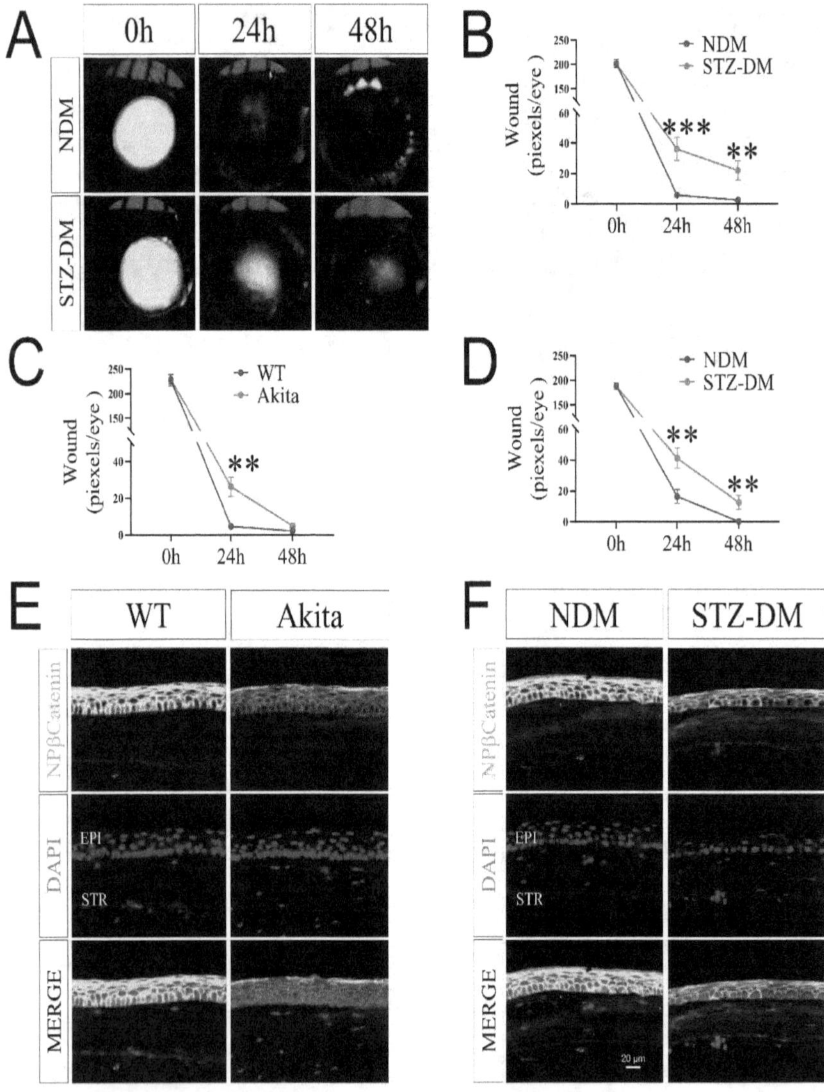



**Figure 2.3 Comparison of corneal wound healing rates of diabetic (DM) animal models and non-diabetic (NDM) control.**
(A) Representative fluorescence staining images showing corneal wounds in STZ-induced DM mice and NDM mice. The post-injury corneas were stained with sodium fluorescein (green) and photographed at indicated time points post-wounding. (B) Quantification of the corneal wound. The progress of wound healing was quantified by measuring wound severity using the pixel of green fluorescence per eye with Image J (n=16). (C) Comparison of corneal wound healing in Akita mice and WT controls (n=5). (D) Comparison of corneal wound healing in STZ-induced

diabetic rats (n=12). (E, F) Representative immunohistochemistry images with an antibody for NP-β-catenin in the corneas 48 hr post-wounding from 5-month-old Akita mice and STZ-induced diabetic mice (3 months of diabetes) and their respective NDM controls (n=5). Scale bars, 20 μm. All values are mean ± SEM. **P<0.01; ***P<0.001.

## Corneal wound healing rates correlated with Wnt/β-catenin signaling activities in kallistatin transgenic (KS-Tg) mice

To explore the role of kallistatin and Wnt signaling in cornea wound healing, we used KS-Tg mice. KS-Tg mice showed circulation kallistatin levels 3-fold higher than WT mice, comparable to the increases in diabetic patients (52). Western blot analysis showed that kallistatin levels in the corneas of KS-Tg mice were significantly higher than those of WT controls (Figure 2.4A and 2.4B). As shown by immunostaining (Figure 2.4C) and Western blotting (Figure 2.4D and 2.4E), KS-Tg mice had lower non-phosphorylated β-catenin levels in corneal wound healing compared to WT mice. In addition, the corneal epithelial wound healing rate was significantly lower in KS-Tg mice than in WT mice (Figure 2.4F). Thus, the results suggested that kallistatin expression resulted in lower Wnt/β-catenin signaling in the cornea and delayed corneal wound healing, similar to the phenotype in diabetic mice.

## Local inhibition of the Wnt signaling pathway delayed corneal wound healing

We injected purified recombinant kallistatin protein into subconjunctival space of WT mice to exclude potential impacts of systemic inhibition of Wnt signaling in KS-Tg mice on corneal wound healing, with the same amount bovine serum albumin (BSA) as control. As shown by Figure 2.4G, the recombinant kallistatin protein delayed corneal wound healing compared with the controls.

To further investigate if the regulatory role of kallistatin in corneal wound healing is through the Wnt signal pathway, we injected Mab2F1, a specific LRP6-blocking antibody, into the subconjunctival space of the WT mice, with the same dose of non-specific IgG for control. As shown by Figure 2.4H, subconjunctival injection of Mab2F1 significantly delayed corneal wound

healing relative to the IgG control.

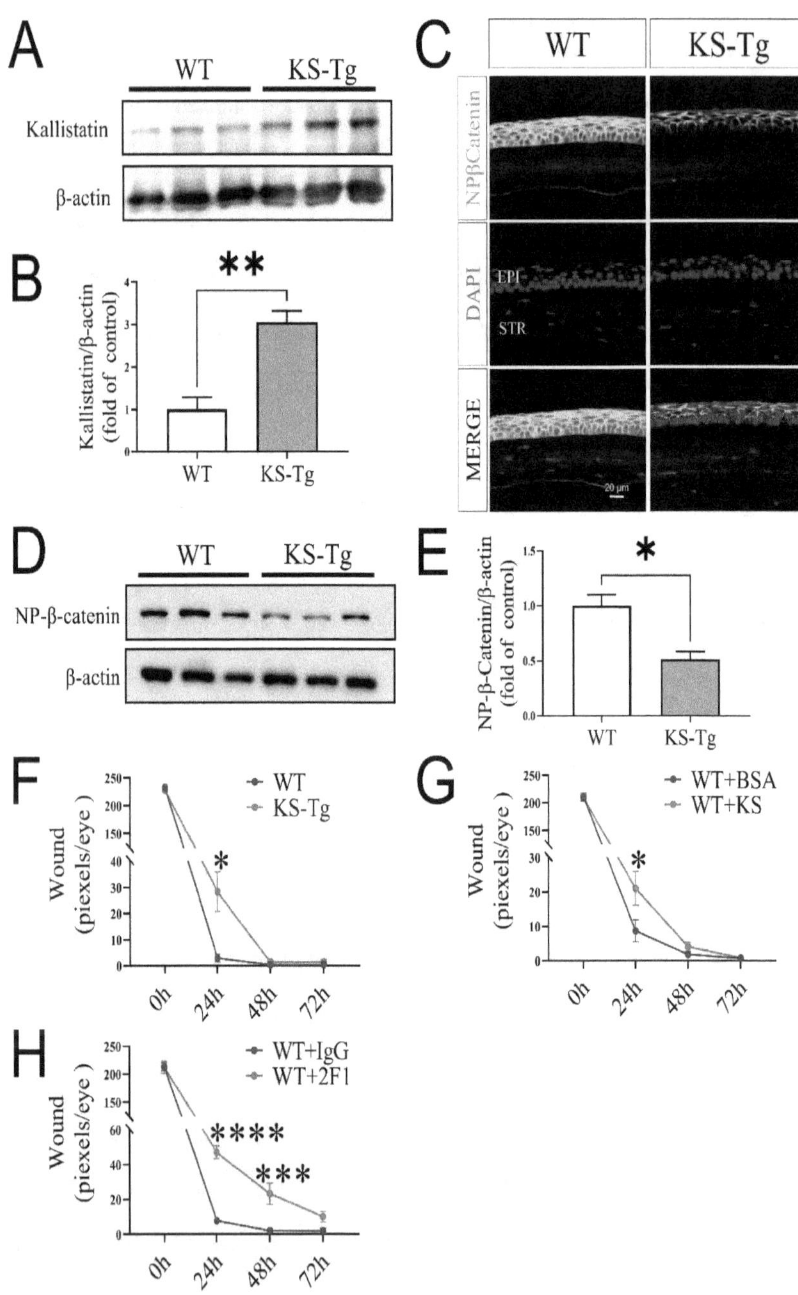

**Figure 2.4 Delayed corneal wound healing in kallistatin transgenic (KS-Tg) mice by inhibition of the Wnt signaling pathway.**
(A) Western blot analysis of kallistatin in the cornea of 5-month-old KS-Tg mice and WT littermates. (B) Densitometry analysis of kallistatin in (A) and normalized by β-actin levels (n=3). (C) Representative images of non-phosphorylated β-catenin (NP-β-catenin) in the corneas of 5-month-old KS-Tg mice and WT littermates. (n=5). (D) Western blot analysis of NP-β-catenin in the corneas. (E) Densitometry analysis of NP-β-catenin in the cornea in (D) and normalized by β-actin levels (n=3). (F) The wound in the cornea from KS-Tg and WT mice was quantified after fluorescein staining using the pixel per eye with ImageJ (n=10). (G) Subconjunctival injection of kallistatin protein (KS, 10 µg/eye) into WT mice, with BSA for control. Wound severity was quantified at post-wounding time as indicated (n=10). (H) WT mice received a subconjunctival injection of 10 µg of Mab2F1 with IgG for control, and then wound severity was quantified at the indicated time points (n=8). All values are mean ± SEM. *P<0.05; ***P<0.001; ****P<0.0001.

**Cornea wound healing rate was promoted in *Vldlr*^-/- mice and suppressed by soluble VLDLR ectodomain**

Our previous study has shown that VLDLR deficiency results in Wnt signaling overactivation in the retina (37; 38; 39). Therefore, we used *Vldlr*^-/- mice for the gain-of-function study of the canonic Wnt pathway activation on corneal wound healing. We measured non-phosphorylated β-catenin levels in the corneas of *Vldlr*^-/- mice. As shown by immunostaining and Western blot analysis, *Vldlr*^-/- mice had higher Wnt/β-catenin signaling activities in the cornea with wound relative to those in the age-matched WT mice with corneal wound (Figure 2.5A-2.5C). In addition, the corneal wound healing assay showed that cornea wound healing was significantly accelerated in *Vldlr*^-/- mice relative to WT mice (Figure 2.5D).

We have identified that the shed soluble VLDLR ectodomain (VLN) can bind to the Wnt co-receptor LRP6 and subsequently inhibit Wnt signaling (38; 109). To determine if the promoted wound healing in the *Vldlr*^-/- cornea results from the over-activation of the Wnt pathway, we subconjunctivally injected adenovirus expressing VLN (Ad-VLN) to *Vldlr*^-/- mice, with adenovirus expressing β-galactosidase (Ad-β-gal) at the same titer as the control. Seven days after the injection, mice received the procedure of epithelial debridement. Ad-VLN significantly delayed the corneal wound closure in *Vldlr*^-/- mice relative to the control virus group (Figure 2.5E). The findings suggested that corneal epithelial wound healing rate highly correlated with Wnt/β-catenin signaling activities in the cornea.

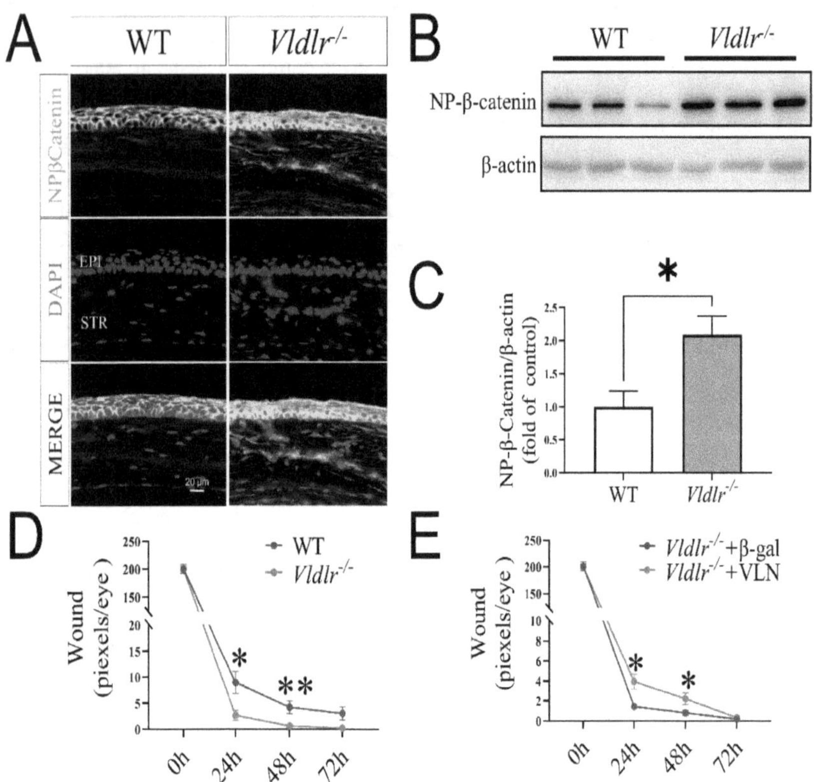


**Figure 2.5 Cornea wound healing rate was promoted in Vldlr-/- mice and delayed by soluble VLDLR ectodomain (VLN).**
(A) Representative immunostaining images of non-phosphorylated β-catenin (NP-β-catenin) (green) and DAPI (blue) in corneal sections of 5-month-old *Vldlr⁻ᐟ⁻* mice and WT littermates (n=5). (B) Western blot analysis of NP-β-catenin in the corneas of *Vldlr⁻ᐟ⁻* mice and WT littermates. (C) Densitometry analysis of NP-β-catenin in the cornea in (B) and normalized by β-actin levels (n=3). (D) The comparison of wound healing progress between *Vldlr⁻ᐟ⁻* and WT mice (n=10). (E) Subconjunctival injection of adenovirus expressing the soluble VLDLR ectodomain (VLN, 10 µl of $1×10^7$ IFU/mL each eye) into *Vldlr⁻ᐟ⁻* mice delayed corneal wound healing compared with adenovirus expressing β-galactosidase (β-gal) control (n=10). All values are mean ± SEM. *P<0.05; **P<0.01.

**Local activation of the Wnt signaling pathway promoted corneal wound healing**

To exclude the potential secondary effect of systemic Wnt signaling changes in *Vldlr⁻ᐟ⁻* mice on corneal wound healing, we subconjunctivally injected adenovirus expressing a constitutively active mutant of β-catenin (Ad-S37A) in which the phosphorylation site Ser37 in β-catenin was substituted by Ala (S37A), into C57BL/6J mice  (33). Adenovirus expressing β-galactosidase (Ad-β-gal) at the same titer was used as control. On the 7th day after the injection, we performed the wound healing assay and found that wound healing was accelerated in the Ad-S37A group relative to the control mice (Figure 2.6A).

Lithium chloride stabilizes β-catenin by inhibiting GSK-3β and is commonly used to activate canonical Wnt signaling intracellularly (34; 35; 36). LiCl (0.9%) was subconjunctivally administered to WT mice with wounded cornea once a day for 3 days. The corneal wound healing in the LiCl-treated group was significantly accelerated (Figure 2.6B).

To determine if Wnt pathway activation intracellular will rescue the delayed healing of corneal epithelial wound in KS-Tg mice, KS-Tg mice received daily subconjunctival injections of LiCl after corneal wounding, with NaCl as control. Our results showed that the corneal wound closure was significantly faster in the LiCl group relative to the NaCl group (Figure 2.6C). This result suggested that activation of Wnt signaling downstream of the kallistatin interaction site will offset its inhibitory effect on wound healing.

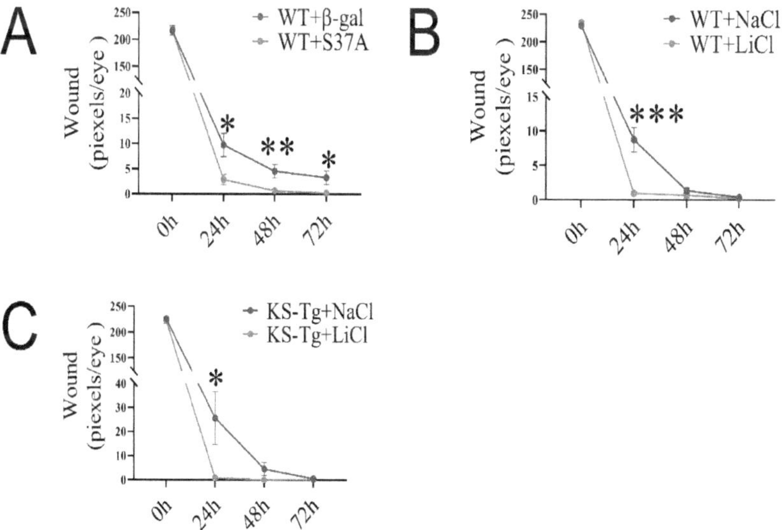


**Figure 2.6 Accelerated wound healing by local activation of the Wnt signaling pathway.**

(A) Subconjunctival injection of a Wnt signaling activator Ad-S37A (10 µl of 1×10$^7$ IFU/mL per eye) enhanced corneal wound closure in WT mice, relative to the control injected with the same titer of Ad-β-gal (n=10). (B) WT mice receiving LiCl (10 µl of 0.9% per eye) subconjunctival injection with NaCl for control (n=10). (C) KS-Tg mice receiving LiCl (10 µl of 0.9% per eye) subconjunctival injection with NaCl as control (n=10). All values are mean ± SEM. *P<0.05; **P<0.01; ***P<0.001.

## EGFR expression levels were upregulated by Wnt/ β-catenin signaling in the corneas

As shown by Western blot analysis, non-phosphorylated β-catenin levels in the cornea with wound were significantly lower in Akita mice and STZ-induced diabetic mice than their age-matched non-diabetic controls (Figure 2.7A and 2.7B). In addition, reduced EGFR expression levels were demonstrated in diabetic mouse corneas, correlating with lower Wnt/β-catenin signaling activities (Figure 2.7A and 2.7B). Inhibition of Wnt/β-catenin signaling in the cornea by subconjunctival injection of the Wnt signaling blocking antibody, Mab2F1, downregulated the expression of EGFR (Figure 2.7C), while Ad-S37A substantially promoted the expression of EGFR (Figure 2.7D).

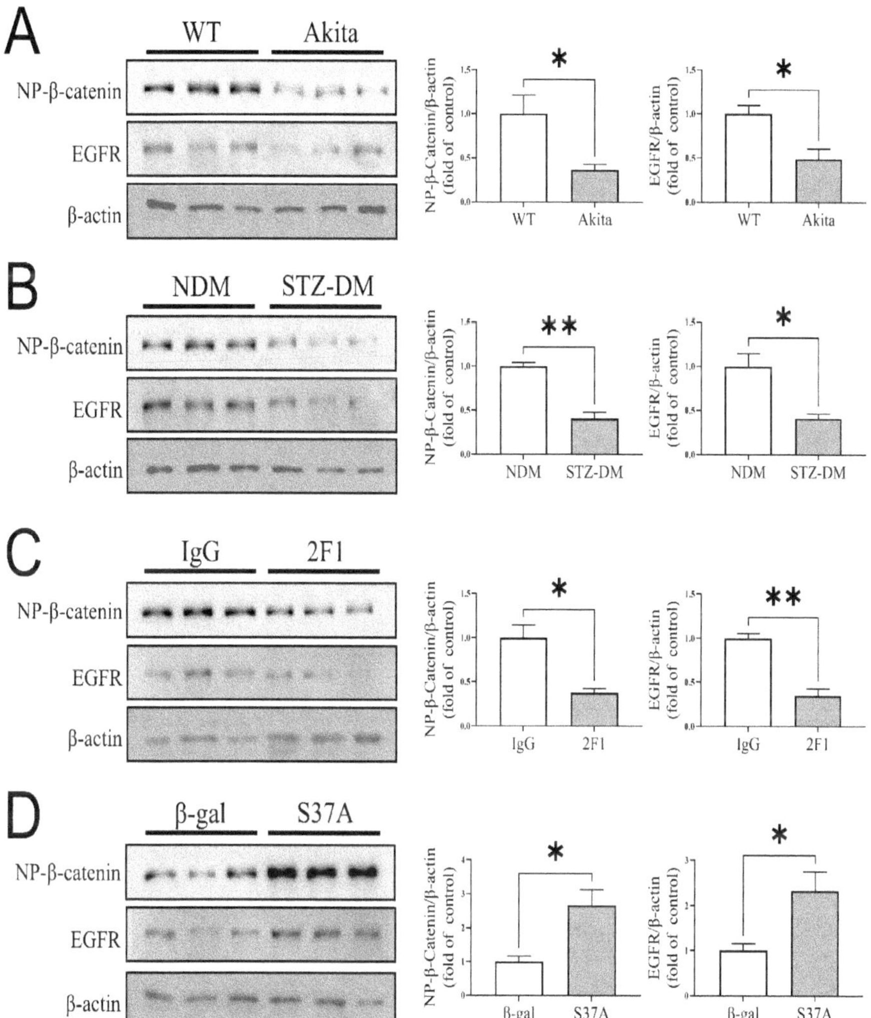

**Figure 2.7 EGFR expression levels were associated with Wnt/β-catenin signaling in the corneas.**

Representative Western blot for non-phosphorylated β-catenin (NP-β-catenin) and EGFR and densitometry quantification in the corneas from 5-month-old Akita mice (A), STZ-induced DM mice (B), WT mice with a subconjunctival injection of Mab2F1 (C) and Ad-S37A (D) and their respective controls. Values are mean ± SEM (n=3). *P<0.05; **P<0.01.

**Kallistatin blocked Wnt signaling-enhanced HCEC proliferation and migration in a concentration-dependent manner**

Epithelial cell proliferation and migration are key steps during the corneal wound healing process (8; 110). To establish the direct effect of Wnt signaling on corneal epithelial cells, we evaluated the proliferation and migration of cultured primary HCEC treated with Wnt3a conditioned medium (WCM), with L cell-conditioned medium (LCM) as control. As shown in Figures 2.8A and 2.8B, WCM stimulated HCEC proliferation and migration. In contrast, kallistatin suppressed the HCEC proliferation and migration induced by WCM in a concentration-dependent manner. In correlation with this effect, Western blot analysis showed that kallistatin downregulated non-phosphorylated β-catenin and EGFR levels in HCEC (Figure 2. 8C and 2.8D), further confirming the *in vivo* findings.

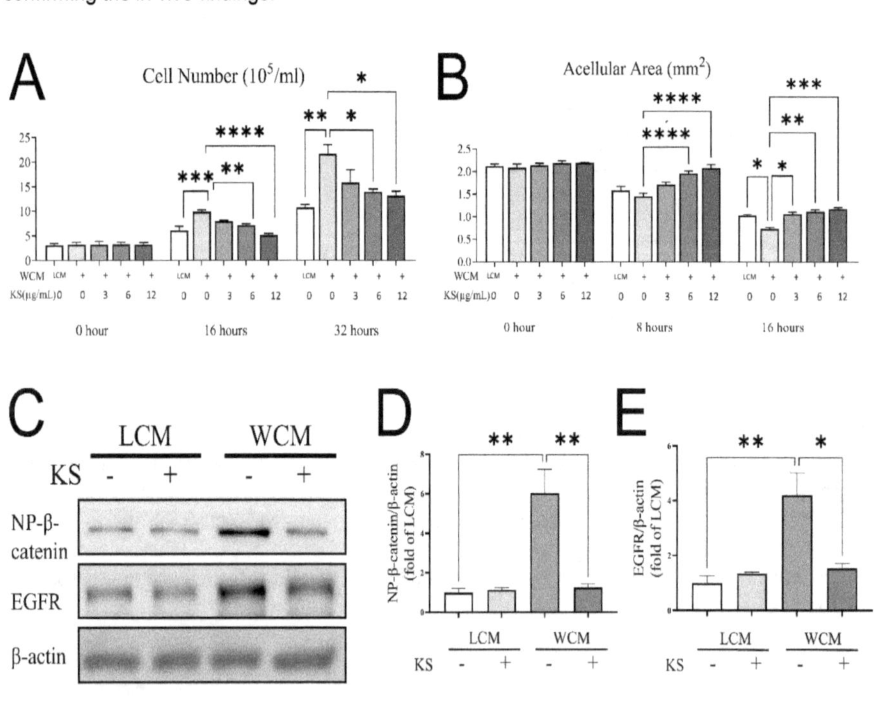

**Figure 2.8 Effect of kallistatin on human corneal epithelial cells (HCEC).**
(A) HCEC were treated with 20% L cell-conditioned medium (LCM) or Wnt3a conditioned medium (WCM) with or without different concentrations of human kallistatin as indicated. Viable cells were quantified at 0, 16, 32 hr (n=3-6). (B) HCEC were treated with WCM and various concentrations of kallistatin after 100% confluence. *In vitro* "wound" was created then 6 images of each scratch

were captured at the indicated time points. The acellular area was measured by ImageJ (n=5). (C) Representative Western blots of non-phosphorylated β-catenin (NP-β-catenin) and EGFR in HCEC with indicated treatment. HCEC were treated with 20% LCM or WCM with or without 12 µg/mL kallistatin for 48 hr. (D, E) Protein levels of NP-β-catenin and EGFR in (C) were quantified by densitometry (n=3). Values are mean ± SEM. *P<0.05; **P<0.01; ***P<0.001; ****P<0.0001.

## DISCUSSION

Increasing evidence suggests that various corneal components (epithelium, stroma, nerves, and endothelium) are affected by diabetes (111; 112). Delayed corneal epithelial wound healing may lead to sight-threatening complications, including ocular surface irregularities, microbial keratitis and corneal scarring (93). However, the molecular mechanism for the diabetes-induced corneal wound healing deficiency remains elusive.

Numerous studies have confirmed that the Wnt/β-catenin signaling pathway is essential for cell proliferation, differentiation and migration (29; 113; 114; 115). Using Wnt activators and inhibitors, the present study provided evidence supporting that canonical Wnt signaling plays an important role in corneal wound healing, and diabetes suppressed Wnt signaling in the cornea, which represents a mechanism for the impaired cornea wound healing in diabetes. Toward the mechanism for the dysregulation of Wnt signaling in diabetic cornea, we found kallistatin, an endogenous inhibitor of Wnt signaling, is upregulated in the diabetic cornea. High levels of kallistatin alone are sufficient to suppress Wnt signaling and delay corneal wound healing, suggesting that diabetes-induced increases of kallistatin suppress cornea epithelial wound healing in diabetes through Wnt/β-catenin signaling. Our results also suggest that the Wnt signaling pathway promotes wound healing at least in part through upregulation of EGFR expression in corneal epithelial cells. These results provided *in vivo* and *in vitro* evidence indicating that elevated levels of kallistatin in diabetic cornea contribute to cornea wound healing delay by suppressing Wnt signaling activation. These findings provided new insights into the regulation of cornea wound healing, which has the potential to contribute to the development of new therapeutic strategies for impaired corneal wound healing in diabetes.

β-catenin is an essential effector of the canonical Wnt pathway (31). In the present study, we identified increased non-phosphorylated β-catenin levels in the wounded cornea. To verify Wnt signaling activation during wound healing, we also measured β-catenin activity using Axin2-lacZ mice, a commonly accepted Wnt reporter model. The results confirmed the increased Wnt pathway activation during the epithelial wound healing process. Limbal stem cells (LSCs) located at the corneoscleral junction play an essential role in corneal epithelium renewal and corneal wound healing (116; 117; 118). As shown by X-gal staining, Wnt signaling is activated in the limbus area and peripheral cornea during wound healing, suggesting that Wnt signaling activation in LSCs may contribute to the corneal epithelial repair. Furthermore, accumulating evidence has shown that Wnt signaling may actively participate in stem cell self-renewal and differentiation (119; 120; 121). Whether targeting the Wnt pathway in LSCs directly has therapeutic potential for cornea wound healing requires further investigation.

The mechanism by which Wnt/β-catenin signaling regulates corneal wound repair is not entirely understood. The canonical Wnt signal activation causes an accumulation of non-phosphorylated β-catenin in the cytoplasm and its eventual translocation into the nucleus to act as a transcription factor (31). β-catenin activates expression of a number of growth factors and their receptors (30; 122), which regulate cell growth, proliferation, migration, differentiation, and adhesion during wound healing (8). EGFR is one of the target genes regulated by Wnt/β-catenin signaling in multiple tissues (123; 124; 125). Wnt ligands have been shown to activate EGFR signaling which increases the proliferation and invasion of fibroblast and glioma cells (126; 127). Consistently, we found that EGFR is upregulated in corneal cells by Wnt signaling, which represents a mechanism for Wnt signaling to promote corneal epithelial cell proliferation and wound healing. Nakamura et al. reported that EGFR inhibition affects epithelial cell proliferation and stratification during corneal epithelial wound healing (128).

In this study, we found that wound-induced Wnt signaling activation was significantly suppressed in diabetic mouse corneas. The causes of suppressed Wnt signaling in diabetic cornea were not yet known. We previously found that serum kallistatin levels are increased in the circulation of diabetic patients, which may contribute to impaired skin wound healing through blocking LRP6, an essential co-receptor in the Wnt/β-catenin pathway (52; 102). Here, we found for the first time that levels of kallistatin were increased in the corneas from human donors with diabetes, compared to subjects without diabetes. To define the role of the diabetes-induced increases of kallistatin levels in corneal wound healing deficiency, we used kallistatin transgenic mice and showed that elevated levels of kallistatin alone in non-diabetic KS-TG mice resulted in delayed corneal wound healing, recapitulating phenotypes of the diabetic cornea. We also found that local application of kallistatin alone delayed mouse corneal wound closure. Also, *in vitro* study revealed that kallistatin significantly suppressed HCEC proliferation and migration induced by Wnt ligand in a concentration-dependent manner. These *in vivo* and *in vitro* results confirmed that kallistatin directly acted on the Wnt signal pathway in cornea epithelial cells and delayed corneal wound healing. Subconjunctival injection of kallistatin protein alone is sufficient to delay corneal wound healing. Consistently, activation of Wnt signaling at the β-catenin level, downstream of the kallistatin binding site, offset the inhibitory effect of kallistatin on HCEC proliferation. Taken together, these observations suggest for the first time that the increased levels of kallistatin in the diabetic cornea are responsible, at least in part, for the Wnt signaling inhibition in the cornea, leading to delayed corneal wound healing in diabetes. Therefore, these findings suggest that diabetes-induced upregulation of kallistatin levels contributes to DK and represents a potential drug target.

Previously, we have found that VLDLR inhibits Wnt signaling by dimerizing with LRP6 through its extracellular domain (VLN) (39; 109). Further, we have shown that VLN is naturally shed into the extracellular space, to function as a soluble Wnt inhibitor (39). However, the function of VLDLR in the cornea has not been carefully studied. The present study demonstrated that Wnt signaling is overactivated in the cornea of *Vldlr*[-/-] mice, suggesting that VLDLR also regulates Wnt signaling in the cornea. In consistent, corneal wound healing is enhanced in *Vldlr*[-/-] mice. Since the full-length VLDLR also has other functions such as lipid transport and metabolism, *Vldlr*[-/-] mice manifested a disturbed lipid profile. To exclude possible impacts of the systemic lipid disturbance, we overexpressed VLN locally using adenovirus vector subconjunctival injection. The local expression of VLN alone impaired corneal wound healing, further supporting that impact of VLDLR on wound healing is through regulation of Wnt signaling in the cornea. To verify the impacts of Wnt inhibition on wound healing, we also injected a monoclonal antibody Mab2F1 that specifically binds to LRP6, blocking Wnt signaling activation (32). Consistent with VLN, this specific Wnt blocking antibody also delayed corneal wound healing.

To further define the cell target of Wnt regulation, we used cultured primary human corneal epithelial cells. Wnt activation by Wnt ligand indeed promoted migration and proliferation of corneal epithelial cells. Consistent with the *in vivo* observation, kallistatin blocked Wnt signaling in these cells, subsequently downregulating EGFR expression and inhibiting proliferation and migration of cornea epithelial cells. Therefore, it is plausible to suggest that upregulation of EGFR in epithelial cells may represent a mechanism for the function of Wnt signaling in promoting wound healing.

Lithium activates Wnt singling at the $GSK3\beta$ level (129). Our results demonstrated that activation of Wnt signaling downstream of LRP6 by lithium offsets the inhibitory effect of kallistatin, which blocks LRP6, on corneal wound healing in KS-Tg mice. Furthermore, *in vitro* study showed that activation of Wnt signaling alone by Wnt ligand promoted HCEC proliferation and migration, suggesting that Wnt signaling directly targets corneal epithelial cells and promotes epithelial wound repair. Our findings suggested that early local modulation of kallistatin/Wnt/$\beta$-catenin activities may benefit the management of diabetic corneal complications.

Wnt signaling regulation is a complex process. It has been well established that Wnt signaling is overactivated in the retina and kidney of diabetic animal models, contributing to diabetic retinopathy and nephropathy (31; 130). In contrast, the Wnt pathway is suppressed in the skin under diabetes, which plays a role in impaired skin wound healing in diabetes (52). The present study demonstrated that Wnt signaling is down-regulated in the diabetic cornea, a change similar to that in the diabetic skin. It remains to be studied how diabetes confers the differential regulation of Wnt signaling in different tissues.

In conclusion, the present study identified that diabetes-induced kallistatin overexpression may be responsible, at least in part, for the deficient cornea wound healing through suppression of Wnt signaling in diabetic cornea. Further studies are warranted to determine if inhibition of kallistatin or activation of Wnt signaling in the cornea may have therapeutic potential in DK.

**CHAPTER III**

**PEROXISOME PROLIFERATOR-ACTIVATED RECEPTOR-A (PPARA) REGULATES**

**WOUND HEALING AND MITOCHONDRIAL METABOLISM IN THE CORNEA**

The chapter that follows is an adaptation from a manuscript titled "Peroxisome Proliferator-Activated Receptor-α (PPARα) Regulates Wound Healing and Mitochondrial Metabolism in the Cornea", published in the Journal *Proceedings of the National Academy of Sciences (PNAS)*. Wentao Liang and Li Huang performed experiements in Figures 3.1B-M, 3.2C, 3.3C-G, and 3.4C-G. The data in Figure 3.1A were generated by Amy Whelchel and Wentao Liang. Tian Yuan performed the assay in Figure 3.2A and 3.5S. Wentao Liang acquired and analyzed the results in the remaining figures. The experimental animals in Figures 3.1B-M, 3.2B-F, and 3.3A-H were provided by Xiang Ma and Rui Cheng. The manuscript was written by Wentao Liang and Li Huang. The research was designed, and the data were analyzed by Yusuke Takahashi, Dimitrios Karamichos, and Jian-Xing Ma. The manuscript was also reviewed and edited by the authors mentioned above. Citation: "Liang W, Huang L, Whelchel A, Yuan T, Ma X, Cheng R, Takahashi Y, Karamichos D, Ma JX. Peroxisome proliferator-activated receptor-α (PPARα) regulates wound healing and mitochondrial metabolism in the cornea. *Proc Natl Acad Sci U S A*. 2023 Mar 28;120(13):e2217576120. doi: 10.1073/pnas.2217576120. Epub 2023 Mar 21." The electronic version: https://www.pnas.org/doi/10.1073/pnas.2217576120.

# ABSTRACT

Diabetes can result in impaired corneal wound healing. Mitochondrial dysfunction plays an important role in diabetic complications. However, the regulation of mitochondrial function in diabetic cornea and its impacts on wound healing remain elusive. The present study aimed to explore the molecular basis for the disturbed mitochondrial metabolism and subsequent wound healing impairment in diabetic cornea. Seahorse analysis showed that mitochondrial oxidative phosphorylation is a major source of ATP production in human corneal epithelial cells. Live cornea biopsy punches from type 1 and type 2 diabetic mouse models showed impaired mitochondrial functions, correlating with impaired corneal wound healing, compared to non-diabetic controls. To approach the molecular basis for the impaired mitochondrial function, we found that Peroxisome Proliferator-Activated Receptor-α (PPARα) expression was downregulated in diabetic human corneas. Even without diabetes, global *PPARα* knockout mice and corneal epithelium-specific *PPARα* conditional knockout mice showed a disturbed mitochondrial function and delayed wound healing in the cornea, similar to that in diabetic corneas. In contrast, fenofibrate, a PPARα agonist, ameliorated mitochondrial dysfunction and enhanced wound healing in the corneas of diabetic mice. Similarly, corneal epithelium-specific *PPARα* transgenic overexpression improved mitochondrial function and enhanced wound healing in the cornea. Furthermore, PPARα agonist ameliorated the mitochondrial dysfunction in primary human corneal epithelial cells exposed to diabetic stressors, which was impeded by siRNA knockdown of *PPARα*, suggesting a PPARα-dependent mechanism. These findings suggest that downregulation of PPARα plays an important role in the impaired mitochondrial function in the corneal epithelium and delayed corneal wound healing in diabetes.

**SIGNIFICANCE STATEMENT**

Diabetic keratopathy (DK) is a common diabetic complication and can impair corneal wound healing. DK lacks effective therapy as its pathogenesis is unclear. In this work, we identified for the first time that human corneal epithelial cells utilize mitochondrial oxidative phosphorylation as a major source of ATP production. In addition, we identified PPARα as a key regulator of mitochondrial function in the cornea and found that diabetes-induced PPARα downregulation plays a pathogenic role in mitochondrial dysfunction and impaired wound healing in the cornea. These findings identified a new function of PPARα in the cornea and revealed a new pathogenic mechanism for diabetes-induced corneal wound healing delay. Further, these results suggest that PPARα agonist has therapeutic potential for DK.

**INTRODUCTION**

Diabetes Mellitus (DM) is a metabolic disease, which can lead to a number of complications including chronic kidney disease, nerve damage, and other problems with feet, vision, and mental health (2; 131; 132; 133; 134). Diabetic corneal complications including corneal nerve degeneration, wound healing delay and ulcer occur in more than half of diabetic population (7; 17; 28). Despite extensive research, diabetic cornea lacks effective treatment, and the pathogenesis for the corneal defects induced by diabetes is not fully understood.

Growing evidence has shown that mitochondrial dysfunction is closely associated with diabetic complications (135; 136; 137). However, the direct impact of diabetes on corneal metabolism is unclear, representing a significant knowledge gap. The metabolic profiles of corneal cells in diabetes and their regulation have not been previously investigated. The molecular basis underlying impaired wound healing in diabetic cornea has not been well understood.

Peroxisome Proliferator-Activated Receptor-α (PPARα) was originally known to regulate lipid metabolism in the liver (65). Its agonists are clinically used for the treatment of dyslipidemia (138; 139; 140). More recently, PPARα agonist fenofibrate has been reported to have robust therapeutic effect on diabetic retinopathy in type 2 diabetic patients (141; 142). Our recent study demonstrated, for the first time, that PPARα is expressed at high levels in the cornea, particularly in epithelial cells, and *PPARα* knockout (KO) alone resulted in spontaneous corneal nerve degeneration, epithelial erosion, and impaired corneal sensitivity, closely recapitulating pathologies seen in diabetic keratopathy (DK) in diabetic patients (75). In addition, our previous study showed that PPARα is critical for neuronal survival and energy metabolism in the retina (143). Despite these findings, the role of PPARα in the regulation of corneal cell metabolism and cornea wound healing has not yet been explored.

In the present study, we compared the metabolic profiles of primary human corneal stromal fibroblasts and epithelial cells utilizing a Seahorse XFe96 Analyzer. We determined the role of PPARα in the regulation of mitochondrial function and wound healing in the cornea using *PPARα*$^{-/-}$ mice, corneal epithelium-specific *PPARα* conditional KO mice and transgenic mice. The present study also explored therapeutic potential of PPARα agonist on wound healing deficiency in diabetic cornea.

## MATERIALS AND METHODS

### Ethical approval and informed consent

The study adhered to the tenets of the Declaration of Helsinki and was performed with the Institutional Review Board (IRB) approval from the University of Oklahoma Health Sciences

Center (IRB protocol #3450). Donor eyes from patients with diabetes and non-diabetic controls were obtained from Lions Gift of Sight Eye Bank (Saint Paul, MN). All methods were performed in accordance with federal and institutional guidelines and all human samples were de-identified prior to analysis.

**PPARα RNAscope *in situ* hybridization**

Human donor eyes dissected within 12 hr postmortem were immediately preserved in Davidson's fixation solution for 24 hr and then transferred to 10% buffered formalin for storage and paraffin section. Human PPARα fluorescent *in situ* hybridization was performed using the RNAscope Multiplex Fluorescent V2 Assay kit (Advanced Cell Diagnostics #323110 and #445201; Santa Ana, CA) according to the manufacturer's instruction. Negative control assays were conducted using a 3-plex negative control probe provided by the manufacturer (Advanced Cell Diagnostics #320871). *In situ* hybridization was followed by DAPI staining, and then fluorescent signals were photographed under an Olympus laser scanning confocal microscope (FV1200; Bartlett, TN). The total number of PPARα mRNA puncta in the corneal epithelium was counted by ImageJ (National Institutes of Health, Bethesda, MD) and normalized by the number of nuclei to quantify the expression of PPARα mRNA.

**Animals**

Male *PPARα⁻ᐟ⁻* mice (20-week-old), wild-type (WT) C57BL/6J mice (8-week-old), Akita (*Ins2^akita*) mice, *db/db* (BKS.Cg-*Lepr^db*/J) mice and their heterozygous littermates in the C57BLKS/J background, were purchased from Jackson Laboratories (Bar Harbor, ME). All experiments were performed following the guidelines of the Association for Research in Vision and Ophthalmology (ARVO) Statement for the Use of Animals in Ophthalmic and Vision Research and approved by the Institutional Animal Care and Use Committee of the University of Oklahoma Health Sciences Center. In all procedures, 50 mg/kg ketamine hydrochloride mixed with 5 mg/kg xylazine (Vedco, Saint Joseph, MO) were used for intraperitoneal injection to anesthetize the mice.

**Corneal epithelium-specific PPARα transgenic mice and PPARα conditional KO mice**

Corneal epithelium-specific Cre transgenic (*Krt12-Cre*) mice were purchased from Jackson Laboratories (stock#023055). PPARα transgenic flox/flox (PCTG) mice which express PPARα under the chicken β-actin promoter upon removal of a floxed stop cassette by desired tissue-specific Cre recombinase were generated through a contract service with Cyagen Biosciences (Santa Clara, CA) following a documented strategy (144). *Krt12-Cre* mice were crossed with PCTG mice to remove of the floxed stop cassette for the generation of *PPARα$^{ECTg}$* mice, which overexpress the PPARα transgene in the corneal epithelium. Overexpression of PPARα in the corneas of *PPARα$^{ECTg}$* mice was verified by immunohistochemistry, in comparison with *Krt12-Cre* mice. *PPARα$^{flox/flox}$* mice in which *PPARα* exon 4 was flanked with loxP sites were generated through a contracted service with Ingenious Targeting Laboratory (Ronkonkoma, NY). To generate corneal epithelium-specific *PPARα* knock-out mice (*PPARα$^{ECKO}$*), *PPARα$^{flox/flox}$* mice were crossbred with *Krt12-Cre* mice, and the KO efficiency of *PPARα* was verified by immunohistochemistry in the corneas of *PPARα$^{ECKO}$* mice relative to those in *Krt12-Cre* mice.

**Streptozotocin (STZ)-induced diabetic mouse model**

As described previously, to induce diabetes, male WT mice (8-week-old) received daily intraperitoneal injections of STZ at a dose of 55 mg/kg for 5 consecutive days (145). Mice with blood glucose levels higher than 350 mg/dL were defined as diabetic animals. The diabetic mice were randomly assigned into two groups: one fed special chow containing 0.014% fenofibrate (LabDiet 5053; TestDiet, Saint Louis, MO) and the other fed regular chow as control for 12 weeks.

**Corneal epithelial debridement wound healing model**

The corneal wound was induced following a documented protocol (105). After mice were anesthetized, an Algerbrush II Corneal Rust Ring Remover (Alloy Medical, San Mateo, CA) was used to create a circular wound of 2-mm in diameter on the central corneal epithelium. The abraded region was stained with 0.1% sodium fluorescein and photographed daily with Micron IV

(Phoenix Technology Group, Pleasanton, CA). The wound area was quantified with ImageJ software.

**Immunohistochemistry of mouse corneas**

The mouse eyeballs were fixed in Davidson's fixation solution for 48 hr for the paraffin section. Following the antigen retrieval with sodium citrate buffer (10 mM sodium citrate, 0.05% Tween 20, pH 6.0) in a steam bath, 3 washes with phosphate-buffered saline (PBS) and blocking with 5% bovine serum albumin (BSA) in PBS, the sections were incubated with anti-PPARα (Novus #NB600-636; Centennial, CO), anti-TOMM20 (abcam #ab186735; Waltham, MA) or anti-nitrotyrosine (abcam #ab61392) antibodies overnight. After 3 washes with PBS, the slides were incubated with Alexa Fluor 488 AffiniPure donkey anti-rabbit IgG (Jackson ImmunoResearch #711-545-152; West Grove, PA) or Alexa Fluor 594 AffiniPure donkey anti-mouse IgG (Jackson ImmunoResearch #715-585-150). The slides were mounted with Vectashield mounting buffer containing DAPI (Vector Laboratories #H-1200; Newark, CA) and photographed under a Zeiss Microscope (Observer Z1; Pleasanton, CA).

**Real-time adenosine triphosphate (ATP) rate assay in cultured cells**

Primary human corneal stromal fibroblasts were isolated from 6 healthy donors (2 females and 4 males whose average age was 41.2 years) by explant culture in EMEM (ATCC #30-2003; Manassas, VA) supplemented with 10% FBS and 1% antibiotic-antimycotic. Upon cell expansion, the cells were passaged and maintained in the same medium for subculture. Primary human corneal epithelial cells (HCEC) from 6 donors (2 females and 4 males, average age 33.5 years) were purchased from ATCC (PCS-700-010) and cultured in medium containing 6.2 mM glucose recommended by the manufacturer (PCS-700-030 and PCS-700-040). Analysis of the metabolic profile in the cells between passages 3-6 was performed using a Seahorse XFe96 Flux Analyzer (Agilent Technologies, Santa Clara, CA). The cells were seeded in a 96-well Seahorse microplate at a density of $5 \times 10^3$ cells/well, and specific compounds including oligomycin (1.5 μM) and a combination of rotenone and antimycin A (RAA, 0.5 µM) were prepared in the cartridge and sequentially injected to measure ATP generation.

**Mitochondrial stress test**

Mice were euthanized with overdose ketamine/xylazine, the whole corneas were isolated, and a 1.5-mm punch biopsy was prepared from the central cornea and loaded into a 96-well spheroid plate with the epithelium side up. Corneal punches were incubated in Seahorse XF base medium (Agilent # 103335-100) supplemented with 10 mM glucose, 1 mM pyruvate and 2 mM glutamine. OCR was measured following the protocol for the mitochondrial stress assay using the Seahorse XFe96 analyzer with sequential injections of oligomycin (1.5 µM), carbonyl cyanide 4-(trifluoromethoxy) phenylhydrazone (FCCP, 2.0 µM), and RAA (0.5 µM). Basal respiration was calculated by subtracting non-mitochondrial respiration from the basal rate prior to injection of oligomycin. Maximal respiration was calculated by subtracting non-mitochondrial respiration from the rate after injection of FCCP.

Primary HCEC were cultured at a density of 5 × $10^3$ cells/well in XF 96-well microplates with/without 4-Hydroxy-2-nonenal (HNE) (EMD Millipore #393204; Burlington, MA) for 24 hr. Hyperglycemic stress was induced by the addition of 23.8 mM of D-glucose (Sigma Aldrich #G7528; St. Louis, MO) for 4 days, and the same concentration of L-glucose (Sigma Aldrich #G5500) was used as a control. Real-time measurement of OCR was recorded with injection of 1.5 µM Oligomycin, 2.0 µM FCCP and 0.5 µM RAA.

**Reactive oxygen species (ROS) assay**

The production of ROS in HCEC was measured using CM-$H_2$DCFDA (Invitrogen #C6827; Waltham, MA) following the protocol of the manufacturer. Following the treatment of the conditioned medium containing HNE/high glucose and fenofibric acid, the cells were washed with PBS and then incubated with CM-$H_2$DCFDA (1:5000 dilution) at 37°C for 30 min. ROS levels were determined by measuring the fluorescence intensity at an excitation wavelength of 483 nm and at an emission wavelength of 530 nm using the Wallac 1420 microplate reader (PerkinElmer Life and Analytical Sciences, Shelton, CT). ROS concentrations were quantified by normalization of the ROS level to the cell protein concentration.

**Western blot analysis**

Western blot analysis was performed as described previously (145). The equal amount of protein was resolved by SDS-PAGE and immunoblotted with primary antibodies for PPARα (Novus #NB600-636), TOMM20 (abcam #ab186735), PGC-1α (Novus #NBP1-04676) and β-actin (Sigma-Aldrich #A5441). Primary antibodies were then detected with HRP-conjugated secondary antibodies (Vector Laboratory #PI-1000 & PI-2000), the band intensity was semiquantified by densitometry using ImageJ software and normalized by β-actin levels.

**Staining of mitochondria and manual scoring of mitochondrial morphology**

HCEC were seeded in 8-chamber culture slides (FALCON #354108; Glendadle, AZ). After treatment, the cells were fixed in 4% PFA for 20 min, washed with PBS containing 0.3% Tween 20 and 0.3% Triton-X-100 for 3 times, then incubated with TOMM20 antibody (abcam #ab186735) at 4 °C overnight. Alexa Fluor 488 AffiniPure donkey anti-rabbit IgG (Jackson ImmunoResearch #711-545-152) was applied for 2 hr and the slides were mounted with Vectashield mounting buffer containing DAPI (Vector Laboratories #H-1200). The cell images were captured under a Zeiss Observer Z1 Microscope and manually classified as "fragmented" if >50% of mitochondrial area consisting of punctiform mitochondria as described previously (146; 147).

**Mitochondrial DNA copy number measurement**

Total DNA was extracted from HCEC using a DNA extraction kit (Zymo Research #D7003; Irvine, CA). The mtDNA levels were measured by qPCR and normalized by nuclear DNA levels as previously described (148). The mtDNA primers used were forward 1 (5'-CACCCAAGAACAGGGTTTGT-3') and reverse 1 (5'-TGGCCATGGGTATGTTGTTA-3') and nuclear DNA primers were forward 1 (5'-TGCTGTCTCCATGTTTGATGTATCT-3') and reverse 1 (5'-TCTCTGCTCCCCACCTCTAAGT-3').

**Mitochondrial membrane electric potential ($\Delta\psi_m$)**

$\Delta\psi_m$ of HCEC was measured using potentiometric dye JC-1 (Invitrogen #T3168) following the protocol of the manufacturer. HCEC were cultured at the condition described above. The cells were stained with 2 µM JC-1 for 30 min and then evaluated for mean cell fluorescence by flow cytometry BD LSRFortessa X-20 Analyzer (Becton Dickinson, San Jose, CA).

**Bromodeoxyuridine (BrdU) cell proliferation**

BrdU Cell Proliferation ELISA Kit (ab126556) from Abcam was used to access cell proliferation rate. Briefly, after incubation with BrdU for 24 hr, the cells were fixed for 30 min. Then, the cells were incubated with an anti-BrdU antibody for 1 hr. Next, peroxidase goat anti-mouse IgG and the HRP substrate was added to the cells and incubated for 30 min. The absorbance was measured at 450 nm using a microplate reader.

**Cell migration assay**

After the cells reached 100% confluence in 12-well plates, a 200 µL sterile pipette tip was used to make a scratch as documented previously (108). The cells were washed twice with PBS to remove floating cells and cultured in treatment media. The scratch acellular area was photographed under Cytation 1 Cell Imaging Multi-Mode Reader (BioTek, Winooski, VT) at two preselected time points (0 and 24 hr). The acellular area was measured using the ImageJ software.

**Transfection of HCEC with siRNA**

PPARα expression was knocked down in HCEC by transfection with the SMARTpool human *PPARα* siRNA (Dharmacon #D-001206-13-20; Boulder, CO) with non-targeting siRNA SMARTpool as control (Dharmacon #D-001810-10-50) using HiPerFect transfection reagent (QIAGEN #301704; Germantown, MD) following manufacturer's instruction.

**Statistical analysis**

Data were presented as mean ± SEM and analyzed by unpaired Student's *t* test for two groups, and ANOVA for more than two groups. $P < 0.05$ was considered statistically significant.

**Data and Resource Availability**

All data are contained within this article. Non-commercial reagents described in this manuscript are available upon request.

64

**RESULTS**

**Distinct metabolic profiles of human corneal epithelial cells and stromal fibroblasts**

To compare the metabolic profiles of human corneal epithelial cells and stromal fibroblasts, ATP production was quantified through real-time measurements of the activity of two main ATP-producing pathways, glycolysis and mitochondrial oxidative phosphorylation in primary human cells. To exclude individual variation of different donors, primary corneal epithelial cells and stromal fibroblasts from six human donors were used to measure ATP production individually, and results were averaged. Seahorse analysis showed that 82.7 ± 1.2% ATP was generated from glycolysis, while only an approximate 17.3 ± 1.2% of total ATP was produced by oxidative phosphorylation in stromal fibroblasts, indicating that stromal fibroblasts strongly favored the glycolysis pathway for energy generation. In contrast, corneal epithelial cells have higher utilization of oxidative phosphorylation as energy source, as approximately 52.0 ± 1.7% of total ATP was generated by oxidative phosphorylation, while 48.0 ± 1.7% from glycolysis (Fig. 3.1A). These data suggested that mitochondrial oxidative phosphorylation is an important source of ATP production in the corneal epithelium which is more susceptible to stress by hypoxia and diabetes.

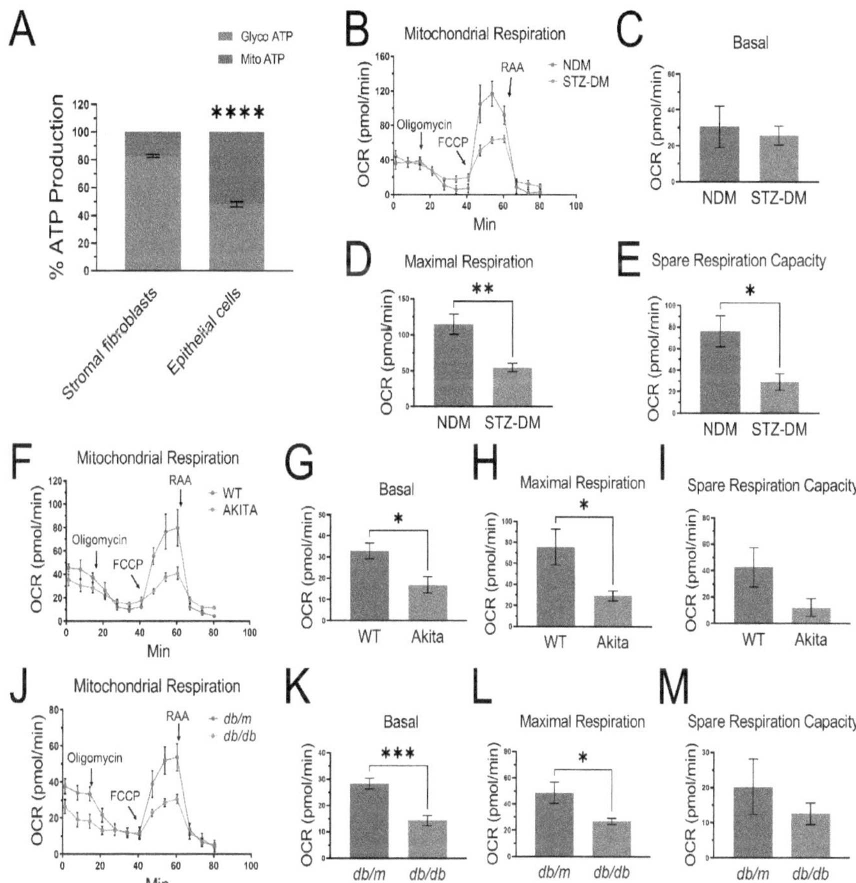

**Figure 3.1 Mitochondrial metabolism is important in the corneal epithelium and is impaired under diabetic condition.**

(A) Real-time ATP rate assay in primary human corneal stromal fibroblasts and epithelial cells ($n$ = 6 donors). In stromal fibroblasts, 82.7 ± 1.2% ATP was generated from glycolysis, while only an approximate 17.3 ± 1.2% of total ATP was produced from oxidative phosphorylation. Corneal epithelial cells have approximately 52.0 ± 1.7% of total ATP production originated from oxidative phosphorylation, with 48.0 ± 1.7% from glycolysis. (B-M) Mitochondrial stress test in the cornea biopsies from STZ-DM mice ($n$ = 6) (B-E), Akita mice ($n$ = 6) (F-I), $db/db$ mice ($n$ = 8) (J-M) and their respective NDM controls. All values are mean ± SEM. *$P$ < 0.05; **$P$ < 0.01; ***$P$ < 0.001; ****$P$ < 0.0001.

## Impaired mitochondrial metabolism in diabetic mouse cornea

To elucidate mitochondrial function changes in diabetic corneas, we measured the OCR using live corneal biopsy punches from type 1 diabetic mouse models (STZ-DM and Akita mice) and a type 2 diabetic mouse model ($db/db$ mice) as well as their respective non-diabetic controls.

Compared to age-matched non-diabetic controls, STZ-DM mice had depressed maximal respiration and spare respiration capabilities in the cornea (Fig. 3.1B-E). Corneas from Akita mice (16-week-old) and *db/db* mice (16-week-old) showed lower basal and maximal OCR than their respective non-diabetic controls (Fig. 3.1F-M). These results suggested that diabetes impaired mitochondrial function in the cornea.

**Decreased PPARα expression in diabetic human corneas**

Previously, we reported that PPARα is expressed in the cornea, and its protein levels are decreased in the corneas of diabetic patients and rats (75). Here, RNAscope assay was used to measure PPARα mRNA levels in the cornea from human donors with diabetes (13 DM, 2 females and 11 males, the average age was 68.3 years), and without diabetes (11 NDM, 5 females and 6 males, the average age was 63.5 years). The result showed that the expression of the PPARα mRNA was downregulated in the corneal epithelium of human donors with DM relative to the non-diabetic corneas (Fig. 3.2A-B).

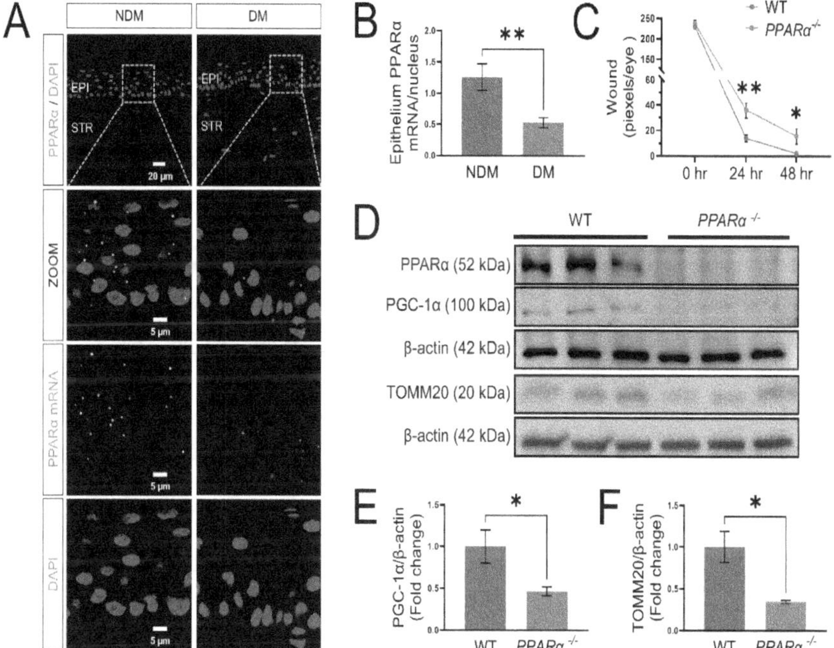


**Figure 3.2 Decreased PPARα levels in diabetic human corneas.**
(A) Representative images of the PPARα mRNA (green) using RNAscope fluorescent assay, with the nuclei counterstained with DAPI (blue) in corneal sections from donors with NDM and DM. EPI, epithelium; STR, stroma. The scale bars represent 20 µm for the upper image and 5 µm for the bottom 3 images. (B) The total PPARα mRNA puncta in the corneal epithelium were counted by ImageJ and normalized by the number of nuclei to quantify the expression of the PPARα mRNA ($n$ of NDM = 11, $n$ of DM = 13). $C$: Wound healing in the corneas from $PPAR\alpha^{-/-}$ and WT mice was quantified after fluorescein staining using the pixel per eye with ImageJ ($n$ = 10). (D-F) Representative Western blots for PPARα, PGC-1α, TOMM20 and β-actin and densitometry quantification in the corneas from 5-month-old $PPAR\alpha^{-/-}$ mice and WT littermates ($n$ = 3). All values are mean ± SEM. $*P < 0.05$; $**P < 0.01$.

**Impaired wound healing and decreased mitochondrial contents in the cornea of $PPAR\alpha^{-/-}$ mice**

To explore the role of PPARα in corneal wound healing and mitochondrial function, we induced corneal epithelial wound in $PPAR\alpha^{-/-}$ mice and their wild-type (WT) littermates. The corneal wound healing was significantly slower in $PPAR\alpha^{-/-}$ mice than that in WT mice (Fig. 3.2C). Western blot analysis showed that levels of mitochondrial marker Translocase of Outer Mitochondrial Membrane 20 (TOMM20) were significantly reduced in the cornea of $PPAR\alpha^{-/-}$ mice at 5 months of age, relative to their WT littermates (Fig. 3.2D, E). In addition, PGC-1α levels in the corneas of *PPARα⁻/⁻* mice were significantly lower than those of WT controls (Fig. 3.2D, F). The results suggested that the ablation of *PPARα* alone resulted in decreased mitochondrial biogenesis and impaired wound healing in the cornea, similar to the phenotypes observed in diabetic mice.

**Activation of PPARα by fenofibrate ameliorated corneal wound healing delay in STZ-DM mice**

Other groups and we demonstrated deficient corneal epithelial wound healing in diabetic animals (145; 149; 150; 151; 152). To explore the role of PPARα in diabetic corneal wound healing, we fed STZ-induced diabetic (STZ-DM) C57BL/6J mice with fenofibrate chow for 3 months starting at the diabetes onset. As shown in Figure 3.3A-C, fenofibrate significantly rescued the expression level of epithelial PPARα and ameliorated the corneal wound healing delay in STZ-DM mice.

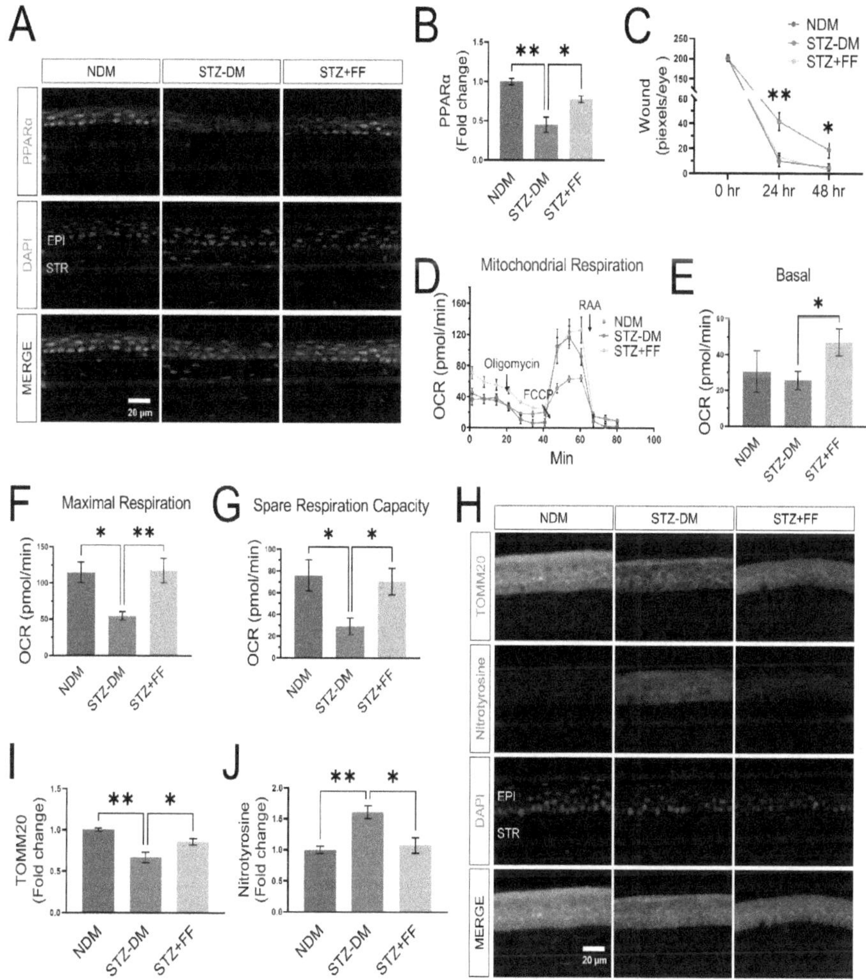

**Figure 3.3 Fenofibrate treatment promoted corneal PPARα expression and prevented mitochondrial function decline in the cornea of STZ-DM mice.**
(A) Representative immunohistochemistry images with an antibody against PPARα (green) in the cornea from non-diabetic mice (NDM), STZ-induced diabetic mice (STZ-DM, 3 months of diabetes) fed with regular chow or chow containing 0.014% fenofibrate (STZ+FF). Scale bars, 20 μm. (B) The intensity of PPARα signals in the epithelial layer in (A) was quantified using ImageJ ($n$ = 3). (C) Quantification of the corneal wound. The progress of wound healing was quantified by measuring wound severity using the pixel of green fluorescence per eye with Image J ($n$ =16). (D-G) Mitochondrial stress test in the corneas from STZ-induced DM mice and NDM controls fed with regular chow or chow containing fenofibrate ($n$ = 6). (H) Representative immunohistochemistry staining images of TOMM20 (green) and nitrotyrosine (red) with the nuclei counterstained by DAPI (blue) in the corneas from NDM mice, STZ-induced diabetic mice with normal chow or fenofibrate chow. (I&J) Immunostaining intensities of TOMM20 ($I$) and nitrotyrosine (J) in the epithelial layer in (H) were quantified using ImageJ ($n$ = 3). All values are mean ± SEM. $*P$ < 0.05; $**P$ < 0.01.

**Fenofibrate prevented corneal mitochondrial dysfunction in STZ-DM mice**

To investigate whether activation of PPARα alleviates metabolic deficiency in diabetic corneas, we measured the real-time mitochondrial respiration using live cornea biopsy punches. The results showed that maximal respiratory rate and spare respiratory capacity were significantly decreased in the corneas of STZ-DM mice, compared to those in age-matched non-diabetic mice. Fenofibrate treatment attenuated the decreases of the basal and maximal respiratory rate and spare respiratory capacity in diabetic mice (Fig. 3.3D-G). To further investigate if fenofibrate also regulates mitochondria content, we measured corneal levels of a mitochondrial protein TOMM20. As shown by immunostaining, TOMM20 levels were significantly reduced in the cornea of STZ-DM mice, relative to the non-diabetic controls, and greatly restored by fenofibrate chow (Fig. 3.3H, I). Increased contents of nitrotyrosine, a marker of reactive oxygen species, were observed in the cornea of STZ-DM mice, which was dramatically attenuated by fenofibrate chow (Fig. 3.3H, J). Taken together, these results indicated that PPARα activation protects corneal mitochondrial function and increases mitochondrion content in diabetic conditions.

**Corneal epithelium-specific *PPARα* KO aggravated mitochondrial dysfunction and corneal wound healing**

To exclude possible secondary effects of systemic hyperlipidemia in *PPARα⁻ᐟ⁻* mice and further substantiate that mitochondria function is regulated by PPARα in the corneal epithelium, we next used a genetic approach. Corneal epithelium-specific *PPARα* KO (*PPARα^ECKO*) mice were generated by crossbreeding *PPARα^flox/flox* mice with corneal epithelium-specific Cre transgenic (*Krt12-Cre*) mice. To achieve corneal epithelium-specific *PPARα* overexpression, the *PPARα* transgene under the chicken β-actin promoter, which is controlled by a floxed stop cassette, was activated by crossbreeding with *Krt12-Cre* mice to generate *PPARα^ECTg* mice. As shown by immunostaining, PPARα expression was suppressed in the corneal epithelium of

*PPARα^ECKO* mice and enhanced in the corneal epithelium of *PPARα^ECTg* mice (Fig. 3.4A, B). *PPARα^ECKO* mice showed delayed corneal wound healing compared to age-matched *Krt12-Cre* littermates, while *PPARα^ECTg* mice had accelerated wound healing (Fig. 3.4C).

To evaluate the role of PPARα expression in mitochondrial function in the corneal epithelium, corneal biopsy punches (1.5-mm diameter) from these mice were used for Seahorse analysis. The mitochondrial respiratory function was significantly reduced in the cornea of *PPARα^ECKO* mice. PPARα overexpression in the corneal epithelium in *PPARα^ECTg* mice greatly promoted the maximal respiration and spare respiratory capacity, compared to *Krt12-Cre* control mice (Fig. 3.4D-G). Immunostaining showed that TOMM20 levels were significantly reduced in the cornea of *PPARα^ECKO* mice and greatly elevated in the cornea of *PPARα^ECTg* mice, relative to the *Krt12-Cre* controls (Fig. 3.4H, I). In addition, nitrotyrosine levels were significantly higher in the corneas of *PPARα^ECKO* mice than those in *Krt12-Cre* controls (Fig. 3.4H, J).

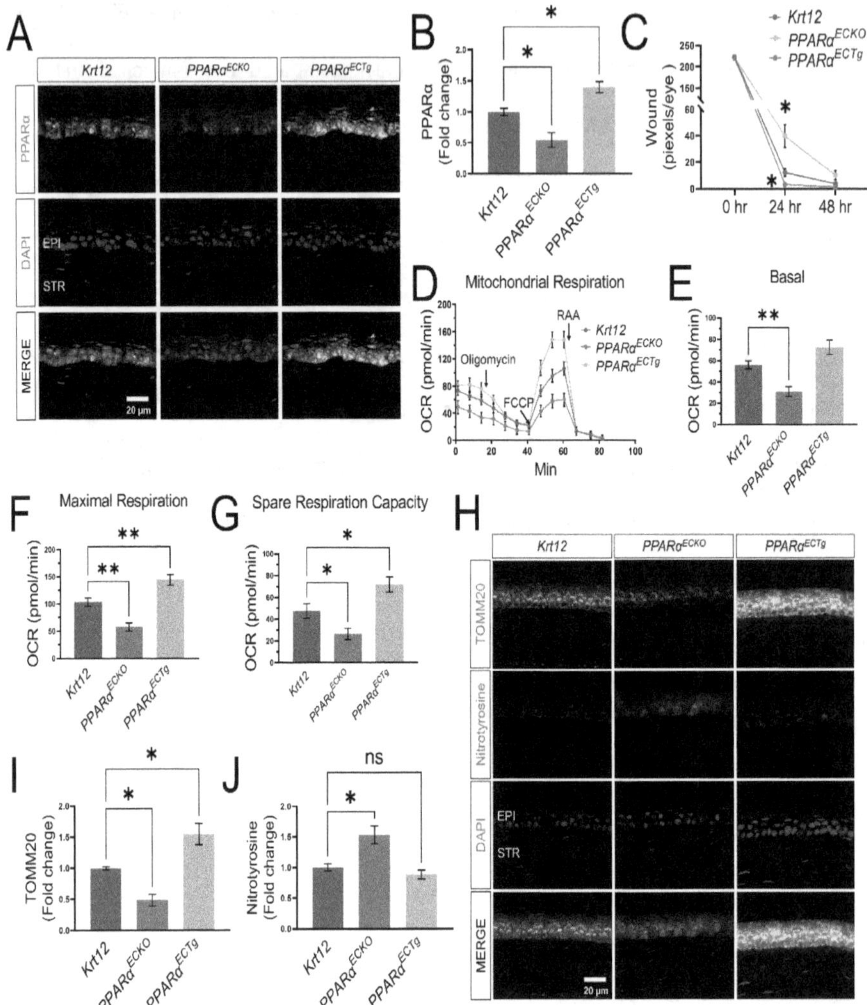

**Figure 3.4 Corneal epithelium-specific *PPARα* KO impaired mitochondrial function and delayed corneal wound healing.**

(A) Representative immunohistochemistry images for PPARα staining (green) in the corneas from *Krt12-Cre (Krt12)*, *PPARα^ECKO* and *PPARα^ECTg* mice. (B) The intensity of PPARα in the epithelial layer in (A) was quantified using ImageJ ($n$ = 3). (C) The corneal wound was quantified after fluorescein staining in *Krt12-Cre*, *PPARα^ECKO* and *PPARα^ECTg* mice and expressed by the pixel per eye with ImageJ ($n$ = 12 - 14). (D-G) Mitochondrial stress test in the corneas from *Krt12-Cre*, *PPARα^ECKO* and *PPARα^ECTg* mice ($n$ = 10). (H) Representative immunohistochemistry images of TOMM20 (green) and nitrotyrosine (red) in the corneas from *Krt12-Cre*, *PPARα^ECKO* and *PPARα^ECTg* mice. (I&J) The intensities of TOMM20 (I) and nitrotyrosine (J) in the epithelial layer in (*H*) were quantified using ImageJ ($n$ = 3). Values are mean ± SEM. *$P$ < 0.05; **$P$ < 0.01; ns, non-significant.

**PPARα agonist treatment ameliorated the mitochondrial integrity damage induced by diabetic stressors in primary human corneal epithelial cells (HCEC)**

To establish the direct effect of PPARα signaling on epithelial cells, we used primary human corneal epithelial cells. HNE is a product of lipid peroxidation and a commonly used stressor of diabetes *in vitro* assays (153; 154; 155). HCEC were also stressed with 30 mM D-glucose (with L-glucose as control) to simulate diabetes stress. Real-Time ATP Rate Assay showed that HNE and high glucose both decreased ATP production from mitochondria in HCEC (Fig. 3.5A-F).

As shown by Western blot analysis, HNE or high glucose exposure decreased the expression of PPARα, PGC-1α as well as TOMM20. Fenofibric acid, an active metabolite of fenofibrate, significantly attenuated the HNE/high glucose-induced downregulation of PPARα, PGC-1α and TOMM20 (Fig. 5G-N). TOMM20 immunostaining showed that HNE and high glucose both increased HCEC with "fragmented" mitochondria, relative to that in controls. Fenofibric acid significantly decreased HNE/high glucose-induced mitochondrial fragmentation in HCEC (Fig. 3.5O-Q).

The mitochondrial DNA (mtDNA) copy number is often used as an indicator of mitochondrial mass (156; 157). The qPCR results demonstrated a significant reduction of mtDNA in HCEC exposed to high glucose, which can be prevented by fenofibric acid (Fig. 3.5R).

The mitochondrial membrane electric potential ($\Delta\psi_m$) of HCEC was evaluated by JC-1 staining and flow cytometry. In healthy cells with a normal $\Delta\psi_m$, the JC-1 dye accumulates in the mitochondria and generates red fluorescence (Q1). In unhealthy cells, the JC-1 enters the mitochondria in a lesser degree and retains the original green fluorescence (Q4) (158). Here, our flow cytometry analysis showed that fenofibric acid treatment group had a higher percentage of Q1 cells, relative to control group (Fig. 3.5S), suggesting that fenofibric acid preserved mitochondrial function in HCEC. After exposure to high glucose, the percentage of low $\Delta\psi_m$ (Q4) in HCEC was increased compared to the control. Fenofibric acid treatment decreased cells with the low $\Delta\psi_m$ under high glucose stress (Fig. 3.5S-T), suggesting that PPARα activation protected

mitochondrial integrity.

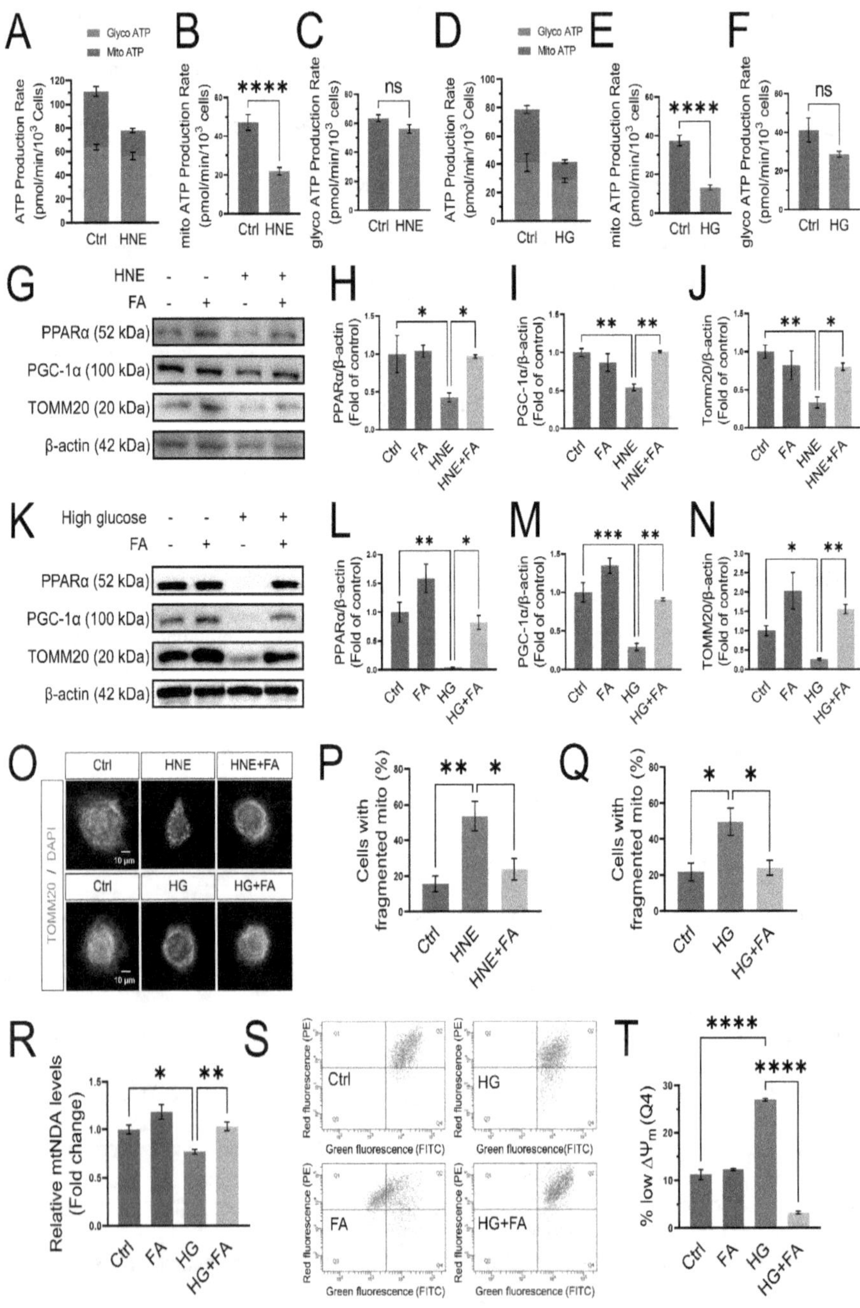

**Figure 3.5 Fenofibric acid treatment ameliorated the impaired mitochondrial integrity induced by diabetic stressor in primary HCEC.**
(A) ATP production from mitochondria and glycolysis was measured using Real-time ATP rate assay in HCEC in the presence or absence of HNE (20 µM) for 24 hr ($n$ = 9). Vehicle (EtOH)-treated cells were used as control (Ctrl). (B&C) Comparison of mitochondrial ATP production rate (B) and glycolysis ATP production rate (C) in panel $A$ ($n$ = 9). (D) ATP production from mitochondria and glycolysis was measured in HCEC exposed to high glucose (HG, 30 mM) for 4 days ($n$ = 6). L-glucose-treated cells (6.2 mM D-glucose and 23.8 mM L-glucose) were used as control (Ctrl). (E&F) Comparison of mitochondrial ATP production rate (E) and glycolysis ATP production rate (F) in panel $D$ ($n$ = 6). (G) Representative Western blots of PPARα, PGC-1α, TOMM20 and β-actin in HCEC exposed to HNE (20 µM) and fenofibric acid (FA, 20 µM) for 24 hr. (H-J) PPARα (H), PGC-1α (I) and TOMM20 (J) in (G) were quantified by densitometry using ImageJ and normalized by β-actin levels ($n$ = 3). (K) Representative Western blots of PPARα, PGC-1α, TOMM20 and β-actin in HCEC exposed to high glucose (30 mM) and FA (20 µM) for 4 days. (L-N) PPARα (L), PGC-1α (M) and TOMM20 (N) in (K) were quantified ($n$ = 3). (O) Representative fluorescence images showing mitochondrial morphology by immunostaining for TOMM20 (green) with the nuclei counterstained by DAPI (blue) in HCEC exposed to HNE (20 µM) or high glucose (30 mM) and FA (20 µM). (P-Q) The percentage of cells displaying a fragmented mitochondria was scored under each condition and averaged in 3 independent experiments. (R) Relative mtDNA levels in HCEC treated with high glucose (30 mM) and FA (20 µM) for 4 days ($n$ = 5). mtDNA content was normalized to nuclear DNA levels. (S) Representative flow cytometry analysis plots showed the distribution of JC-1 stained HCEC exposed to high glucose and FA. (T) The percentage of cells with low $\Delta\Psi_m$ (Q4) was compared between the groups as indicated ($n$ = 3). Values are mean ± SEM. *$P$ < 0.05; **$P$ < 0.01; ***$P$ < 0.001; ****$P$ < 0.0001; ns, non-significant.

**Fenofibric acid treatment ameliorated the mitochondrial dysfunction induced by diabetic stressors, and enhanced proliferation and migration in HCEC**

HNE- and high glucose-treated HCEC showed an increased production of reactive oxygen species (ROS), which was attenuated by fenofibric acid (Fig. 3.6A-B). The mitochondria stress assay showed that fenofibric acid prevented the decreases of basal, maximal respiration and spare respiratory capacity induced by HNE or high glucose in HCEC (Fig. 3.6C-J).

To establish the direct effect of fenofibric acid on corneal wound healing, we evaluated the proliferation and migration of primary HCEC stressed with HNE and treated with fenofibric acid. As shown in Figures 3.6K and 3.6L, HNE suppressed HCEC proliferation and migration, which was significantly alleviated by fenofibric acid treatment. Similarly, high glucose suppressed HCEC proliferation and migration, which was attenuated by fenofibric acid treatment (Fig. 3.6M, N).

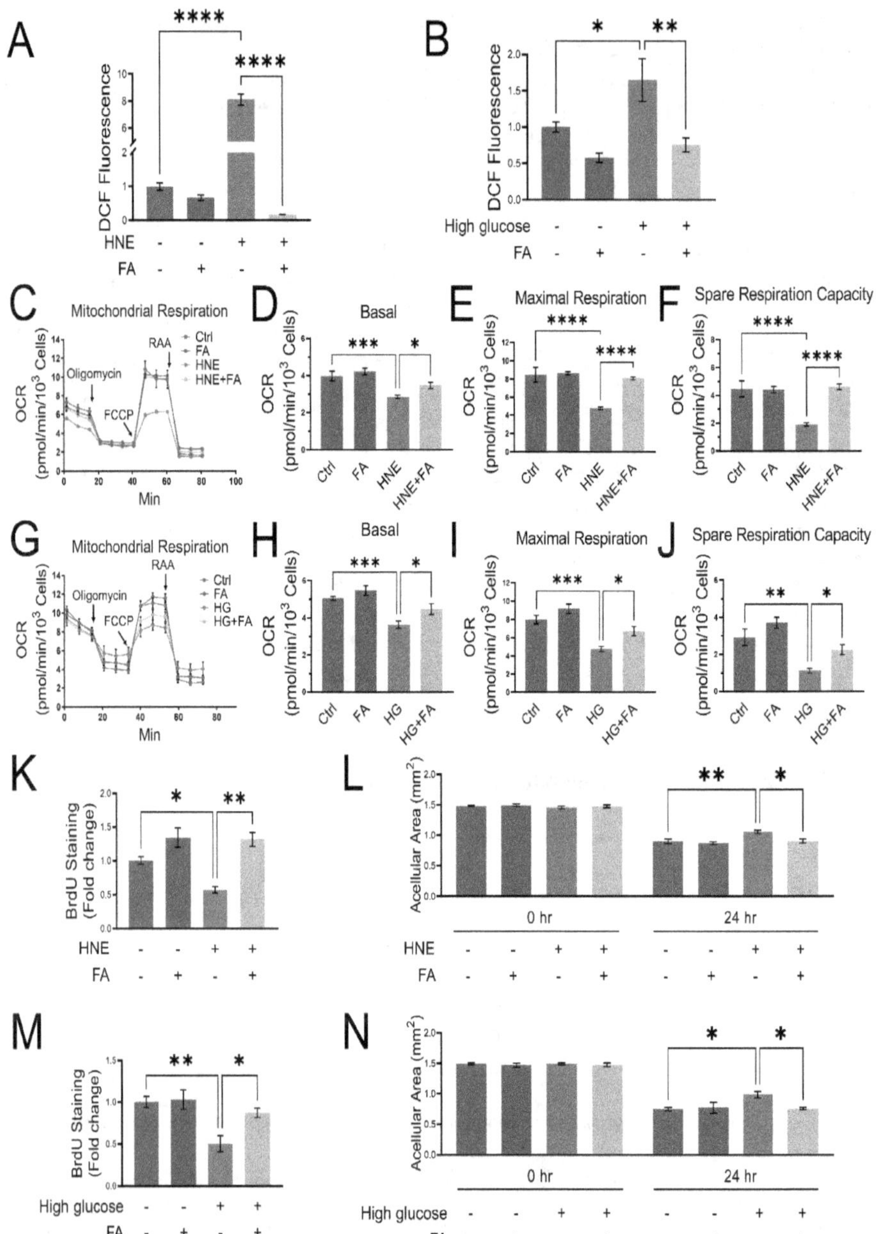

**Figure 3.6 Fenofibric acid treatment ameliorated the mitochondrial dysfunction induced by diabetic stressors, and enhanced proliferation and migration in HCEC.**
*A:* DCF fluorescence signal was measured in HCEC treated with HNE (20 µM) and fenofibric acid (FA, 20 µM) for 24 hr ($n$ = 5-7). *B:* DCF fluorescence signal in HCEC treated with high glucose (30 mM) and FA (20 µM) for 4 days ($n$ = 8). *C-F:* Mitochondrial stress test in HCEC treated with HNE (10 µM) and FA (20 µM) for 24 hr ($n$ = 6-8). *G-J:* Mitochondrial stress test in HCEC exposed with high glucose (30 mM) and FA (20 µM) for 4 days ($n$ = 6). *K:* HCEC proliferation in the

presence or absence of HNE (20 μM) and FA (20 μM) for 24 hr was measured by Cell Proliferation BrdU ELISA ($n$ = 3). *L*: HCEC were treated with HNE (20 μM) and FA (20 μM) after 100% confluence. Images of each scratch were captured after *in vitro* "wound" was created at indicated time points. The acellular area was measured by ImageJ ($n$ = 6). *M-N*: HCEC proliferation ($n$ = 5) and migration ($n$ = 5) were measured after the cells were exposed to high glucose (30 mM) and FA (20 μM) for 4 days. Values are mean ± SEM. *$P$ < 0.05; **$P$ < 0.01; ***$P$ < 0.001; ****$P$ < 0.0001.

**SiRNA-mediated knockdown of *PPARα* aggravated mitochondrial dysfunction in primary HCEC**

To further study the effect of downregulation of PPARα expression on mitochondrial function, HCEC was transfected with a siRNA specific for *PPARα*. Western blotting results confirmed that compared with the scrambled siRNA control group, expression of PPARα was significantly decreased in the cells transfected with the *PPARα* siRNA (Fig. 3.7A, B). Knockdown of *PPARα* suppressed the expression of PGC-1α and TOMM20 in HCEC (Fig. 3.7C, D). The mitochondria stress assay showed that siRNA-mediated knockdown of *PPARα* decreased maximal respiration and spare respiratory capacity in primary HCEC (Fig. 3.7E-H).

Fenofibric acid treatment significantly attenuated HNE- and high-glucose-induced ROS generation in scrambled siRNA-transfected HCEC. However, the effect of fenofibric acid on ROS production was impeded by the siRNA knockdown of *PPARα*, suggesting a PPARα-dependent mechanism (Fig. 3.7I, J).

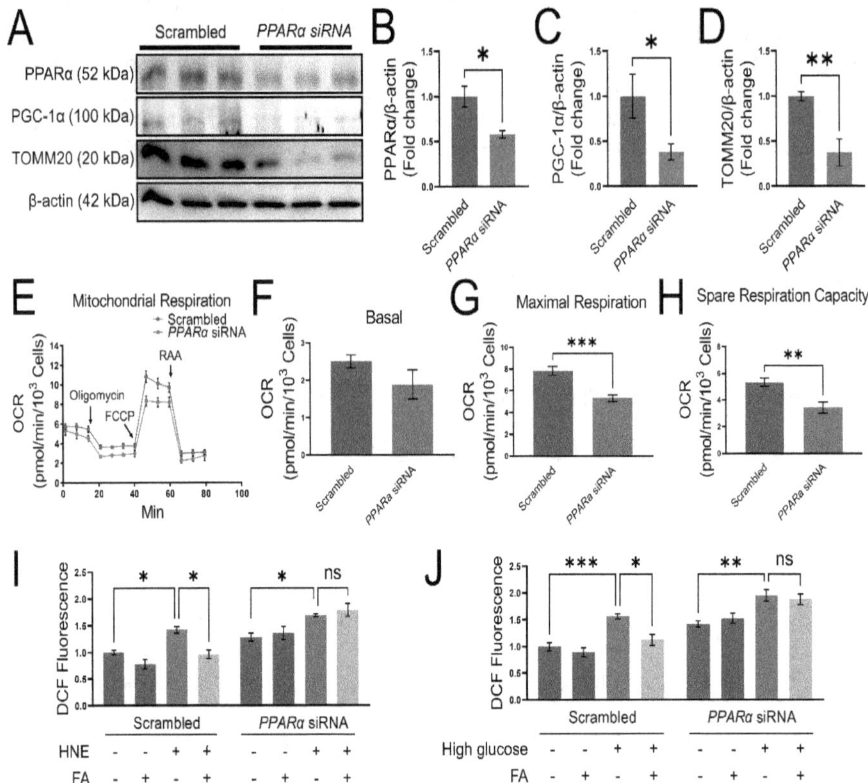

**Figure 3.7 siRNA-mediated knockdown of *PPARα* impaired mitochondrial function in primary HCEC.**
(A-D) Western blot analysis of PPARα, PGC-1α, TOMM20 and β-actin in HCEC transfected with scrambled siRNA or *PPARα* siRNA for 72 hr. Protein levels of PPARα (B), PGC-1α (C) and TOMM20 (D) in panel *A* were quantified by densitometry ($n$ = 3). (E-H) Mitochondrial stress test in the HCEC transfected with siRNA against *PPARα* for 72 hr, with scrambled siRNA as control ($n$ = 6). (I) ROS production was measured in HCEC transfected with scrambled siRNA or *PPARα* siRNA for 72 hr and then exposed to HNE (20 μM) and fenofibric acid (FA, 20 μM) for 6 hr ($n$ = 5-6). (J) After transfection with scrambled siRNA or *PPARα* siRNA, HCEC were exposed to high glucose (30 mM) and FA (20 μM) for 4 days and the ROS production was measured ($n$ = 7). All values are mean ± SEM. *$P$ < 0.05; **$P$ < 0.01; ***$P$ < 0.001; ns, non-significant.

Accumulating evidence suggests that mitochondrial dysfunction plays a key role in the pathophysiology of diabetic complications (135; 136; 137; 159; 160). Corneal wound healing involves epithelial cell proliferation and migration, and requires ATP production. In this study, we found that human corneal epithelial cells use mitochondrial oxidation as a major source of ATP, while cornea stromal fibroblasts predominantly use glycolysis. We also demonstrated declined mitochondrial function in the live cornea punch biopsies of both type 1 and type 2 diabetic mouse models. Furthermore, the present study demonstrated that activation of PPARα alleviated mitochondrial dysfunction and wound healing delay in the diabetic cornea. In consistent, conditional KO of *PPARα* in corneal epithelial cells impaired, while transgenic overexpression of *PPARα* in the corneal epithelium improved, mitochondrial function and wound healing in the cornea. These findings suggest that mitochondrial dysfunction plays a key role in deficiency of corneal wound healing in diabetes, and PPARα is an important regulator of mitochondrial function in the corneal epithelium.

Glycolysis and oxidative phosphorylation are the main sources of ATP production. Only a few early documented studies compared metabolic profiles of the corneal epithelium and stroma (161; 162). It was reported by Langham in 1954, that the acid accumulation rate in the rabbit corneal epithelial layer decreases greatly in the presence of oxygen, while in the stroma the acid production rate is barely changed between the anaerobic and aerobic environment, suggesting that epithelium prefers aerobic environment than stroma (161). In 1985, Greiner et. al found that phosphates associated with energy metabolism were primarily in the corneal epithelium using phosphorus-31 nuclear magnetic resonance (162) and suggested that high-energy phosphate biosynthesis occurs in the corneal epithelium. There was no recent study regarding human corneal metabolic profiles, leaving a major knowledge gap. Here we for the first time compared the metabolic profiles of primary human epithelial cells with those of human stromal fibroblasts side by side. To exclude individual differences from human donors, we used primary corneal epithelial cells and stromal fibroblasts from six different donors and provided the direct evidence showing that mitochondrial oxidation is a major energy source in human epithelial cells by measuring the real-time ATP production. Under the same condition, human stromal fibroblasts predominantly use glycolysis to generate ATP. These results demonstrate that human corneal epithelial cells and stromal fibroblasts have different metabolic profiles, suggesting that regulation of mitochondrial function has a significant impact on epithelial function and wound healing.

Previous studies have suggested that the corneal cells have declined mitochondrial function in diabetes. Mussi et al. showed high glucose culture compromises mitochondrial function in human telomerase-immortalized corneal epithelial cells (84). Aldrich et al. reported that corneal endothelial cells of human donors with advanced diabetes have impaired mitochondrial function as measured by extracellular flux analysis (85). Here, for the first time, we investigated mitochondrial function using live cornea biopsies from both type 1 and type 2 diabetic mice for real-time measurement of mitochondrial function. For the Seahorse analysis, we placed 1.5-mm corneal punches into the plate with the epithelium side on top which are close to the sensor probes of the Seahorse analyzer. Considering that the epithelial cells are more dependent on mitochondria for energy and the epithelium side is closer to the probe, we believe that the OCR measured in corneal biopsies likely reflect the mitochondrial oxidation of the epithelium. The results demonstrated that mitochondrial function was impaired in the corneal epithelium of both type 1 and type 2 diabetic models.

To measure the metabolic activities in isolated corneal epithelium and stroma, we separated the epithelial layer and stroma layer for Seahorse analysis. However, after peeling off the epithelial layer, the mitochondrial function from the isolated epithelial layer or stroma layer became nondetectable by Seahorse assay, suggesting possible damage during the dissection procedure. This represents a limitation of the mitochondrial assay using corneal punches for the Seahorse assay.

To explore the molecular basis for the diabetes-induced mitochondrial function decline in the cornea, we evaluated the role of PPARα. PPARα is a transcription factor that belongs to the nuclear receptor superfamily (62). Upon activation, PPARα heterodimerizes with the Retinoid X Receptor (RXR) and binds to PPAR Response Elements (PPREs) in the promoter regions of target genes including PPARα itself and those involved in many processes such as energy metabolism, oxidative stress, inflammation, circadian rhythm, immune response, mitochondrial genesis and cell differentiation (65; 66; 67; 68; 69; 70; 71). Two independent, prospective clinical studies reported robust therapeutic effects of PPARα agonist fenofibrate on diabetic retinopathy in type 2 diabetic patients (73). Our previous study has shown that diabetes-induced down-regulation of PPARα in the retina plays a key pathogenic role in retinal oxidative stress and inflammation in diabetic retinopathy (74). Recently, we demonstrated that PPARα protein levels are decreased in the corneal epithelium from both type 1 and type 2 diabetic donors compared to non-diabetic human donors (75). *PPARα$^{-/-}$* mice showed  declined corneal nerve densities and increased epithelial lesion in the central cornea (75). It has been reported that PPARα agonist accelerated corneal epithelial healing after alkali injury (76). These observations suggested that PPARα has a role in maintenance of corneal integrity. However, the physiological function of PPARα in the cornea, especially in the regulation of mitochondria function, has not been previously investigated.

To evaluate the impacts of PPARα downregulation on metabolic profile in diabetic cornea, we treated diabetic mice with PPARα agonist fenofibrate. Our results showed that fenofibrate treatment ameliorated mitochondrial dysfunction in diabetic corneas. In consistent, fenofibrate treatment also improved wound healing in diabetic corneas. In contrast, *PPARα KO* alone impaired mitochondrial function and delayed corneal wound healing. Global *PPARα KO* has been shown to result in systemic hyperlipidemia (163). To exclude potential impacts secondary to systemic dyslipidemia in global *PPARα KO*, we generated epithelium-specific *PPARα* conditional KO and transgenic mice for this study. Consistent with the observations from the *PPARα$^{-/-}$* mice, epithelium-specific *PPARα* conditional KO mice also showed impaired mitochondrial function and wound healing delay in the cornea. In contrast, transgenic overexpression of *PPARα* in the epithelium alleviated the mitochondrial dysfunction as well as corneal wound healing delay. These results suggested that epithelial PPARα is important for the regulation of mitochondria function in the cornea.

PPARα is known to regulate PGC-1α (164; 165). PGC-1α plays essential roles in glucose/fatty acid metabolism and mitochondria biogenesis (166; 167; 168). TOMM20, often used as a surrogate of mitochondria mass, is regulated by PGC-1α (167; 168; 169; 170; 171). In this study, we demonstrated that *PPARα* KO mice displayed decreased expression of PGC-1α and TOMM20 in the cornea. To further define the direct effect of PPARα, we treated diabetic mice and cultured primary HCEC with PPARα agonist, fenofibrate or fenofibric acid. Activation of PPARα restored the expression of PGC-1α and TOMM20 in the cornea of diabetic mice. Exposure of primary HCEC to diabetic stressors downregulated the expression of PPARα and impaired ATP production from mitochondria, while glycolysis remained intact. Activation of PPARα using fenofibric acid increased the expression of PGC-1α and TOMM20, and attenuated the decline of proliferation and migration of epithelial cells under diabetic stress. Consistent with the *in vivo* observation in global *PPARα* KO and conditional KO mice, siRNA-mediated knockdown of *PPARα* alone downregulated the expression of PGC-1α and TOMM20 in these cells. Further, mitochondrial fragmentation and mitochondrial membrane electric potential measurements support that diabetic stressor impairs integrity of mitochondria, which can be attenuated by PPARα agonist. Although fenofibric acid is a PPARα agonist, off-target effects were reported (172; 173; 174; 175). Here, we showed that the beneficial effect of fenofibric acid on ROS production was impeded by the PPARα siRNA knockdown, suggesting that fenofibric acid ameliorated epithelial cell mitochondrial function through a PPARα-dependent mechanism. Therefore, it is plausible to suggest that PPARα signaling in epithelial cells may represent an important regulatory mechanism for mitochondrial metabolism and corneal wound healing.

Recent studies have shown that disturbed epithelial-neural-immune cell interactions are a major cause of diabetic neurotrophic keratopathy (2). Our previous study showed that PPARα protects corneal nerve against DM (75). The present study demonstrated that PPARα also promotes corneal epithelial cell proliferation and migration likely through protection of the metabolic function. The regulation of epithelial cell metabolism may also improve neurotrophic environment in the cornea and thus, contributes to nerve protection, which remains to be further investigated.

In conclusion, the present study identified for the first time that PPARα serves as an important regulator of mitochondrial function in the corneal epithelium, and diabetes-induced PPARα down-regulation plays a pathogenic role in wound healing deficiency in diabetic cornea. PPARα has potential to become a new therapeutic target, and fenofibrate may have therapeutic potential in diabetic keratopathy.

**CHAPTER IV**

**A METHOD FOR REAL-TIME ASSESSMENT OF MITOCHONDRIAL RESPIRATION USING MURINE CORNEAL BIOPSY**

The following chapter was adapted from an unpublished manuscript submitted to the Journal *Investigative Ophthalmology & Visual Science (IOVS)* which is under review. Wentao Liang and Li Huang performed experiments, acquired, and analyzed data in Figure 4.1-4.6, and wrote the manuscript. Tian Yuan and Rui Cheng conducted experiments in Figure 4.4A-D and Figure 4.5A-H. Yusuke Takahashi, Gennadiy Moiseyev, Dimitrios Karamichos, and Jian-Xing Ma designed the research, analyzed data, reviewed, and revised the manuscript.

**ABSTRACT**

**Purpose.** To develop and optimize a method to monitor real-time mitochondrial function by measuring the oxygen consumption rate (OCR) in murine corneal biopsy punches with a Seahorse extracellular flux analyzer.

**Methods.** Murine corneal biopsies were obtained using a biopsy punch immediately after euthanasia. The corneal metabolic profile was assessed using a Seahorse XFe96 pro analyzer, and mitochondrial respiration was analyzed with specific settings.

**Results.** Real-time ATP rate assay showed that mitochondrial oxidative phosphorylation is a major source of ATP production in live murine corneal biopsies. Euthanasia methods (carbon dioxide asphyxiation vs. overdosing on anesthetic drugs) did not affect corneal OCR values. Mouse corneal biopsy punches in 1.5-mm diameter generated higher and more reproducible OCR values than those in 1.0-mm diameter. The biopsy punches from the central and peripheral cornea did not show significant differences in OCR values. There was no difference in OCR reading by the tissue orientations (the epithelium side up vs. the endothelium side up). No significant differences were found in corneal OCR levels between sexes, strains (C57BL/6J vs. BALB/cJ), or ages (4, 8, vs. 32 weeks). Using this method, we showed that the wound-healing process in mouse cornea affected mitochondrial activity.

**Conclusions.** The present study validated a new strategy to measure real-time mitochondrial function in live mouse corneal tissues. This procedure should be helpful in studies of the live corneal metabolism in response to genetic manipulations, disease conditions, or pharmacological treatments in mouse models.

# INTRODUCTION

Dysregulated mitochondrial metabolism is imperative in various pathologies, such as metabolic diseases, trauma, and aging (176; 177; 178; 179). Mitochondrial oxygen consumption in freshly isolated mitochondria, cultured cells, or tissues is commonly assessed using a Seahorse Extracellular Flux Analyzer (180; 181; 182). However, the mitochondrial isolation procedure may alter organelle functions by disrupting the cell/organelle structures and intracellular interactions (183). Moreover, *in vitro* measurement using cultured cells could not adequately reflect the *in vivo* status, as tissular/cellular micro-environments and the cell-to-cell interactions may be altered. To overcome this limitation, assessing mitochondrial function in live tissues is of great interest.

Growing evidence has shown that disturbed metabolism plays a key role in the pathophysiology of corneal diseases (184; 185; 186). However, the direct impacts of different disease conditions on corneal mitochondrial metabolism are not fully investigated due to limited methods for measuring metabolism in live corneal tissue. The present study aimed to develop an assay for the real-time measurement of mitochondrial metabolism in live murine corneas.

To investigate the mitochondrial function in live cornea tissues, we developed and validated a new method using a Seahorse XFe96 pro Extracellular Flux Analyzer. We evaluated the impact of different euthanasia methods, punch sizes, and biopsy locations on oxygen consumption rate (OCR). In addition, we compared the corneal OCR values in different sexes, ages, and strains. Altogether, these results will greatly facilitate the study of real-time mitochondrial function in live murine cornea.

METHODS

## Animals

C57BL/6J (#000664) and BALB/cJ (#000651) mice were purchased from Jackson Laboratories (Bar Harbor, ME). All experiments were in adherence to the Association for Research in Vision and Ophthalmology (ARVO) Statement for the Use of Animals in Ophthalmic and Vision Research and approved by the Institutional Animal Care and Use Committee of Wake Forest University School of Medicine.

## Corneal epithelial abrasion

The corneal epithelial wound was induced following a documented protocol (105). Briefly, an ocular burr (Alloy Medical, San Mateo, CA) was used to generate an abrasion on the central cornea after mice were anesthetized by an intraperitoneal (i.p) injection of 50 mg/kg ketamine hydrochloride mixed with 5 mg/kg xylazine (Vedco, Saint Joseph, MO).

## Corneal biopsy preparation

The whole corneas were isolated after mice were euthanized by carbon dioxide asphyxiation or by overdose of anesthetic drug (an i.p injection of 500 mg/kg ketamine and 50 mg/kg xylazine hydrochloride supplement) followed by cervical dislocation. Corneal biopsies prepared using a disposable biopsy punch in 1.0-mm diameter (VWR #33-31AA, Integra LifeSciences, Princeton, NJ) or 1.5-mm diameter (VWR #33-31A) were loaded into a Seahorse XFe96 spheroid microplate (Agilent Technologies, Part# 102978-100, Wilmington, DE) one biopsy per well. Corneal biopsy punches were kept in Seahorse XF base medium (Agilent Part# 103335-100) containing 10.0 mM glucose (Sigma #G7528, St. Louis, MO), 1.0 mM pyruvate (Sigma #S8636), and 2.0 mM L-glutamine (Sigma #G7513) supplement on ice until measurement.

## Real-time adenosine triphosphate (ATP) rate assay

A Seahorse XF real-time ATP rate assay on the corneal biopsy was performed using the Seahorse XFe96 pro Analyzer. The basal OCR was measured first without any added compounds.

Then the OCR was recorded following the injection of oligomycin (Sigma #O4876) at a final concentration of 1.5 µM and a combination of rotenone (Sigma #R8875) and antimycin A (Sigma #A8674) (RAA) at a final concentration of 0.5 µM. For each step (basal, oligomycin, RAA), respectively, the measurement was repeated three times to obtain an average value. Each measurement consisted of three steps: mix for 3 minutes, wait for 0 minutes, and measure for 3 minutes using a sensor cartridge detecting proton production and oxygen levels in each well. The ATP production was calculated with Agilent Seahorse Wave Pro software (version 10.0.1) and Real-Time ATP Rate Assay Report Generator.

**Mitochondrial stress test**

The mitochondrial stress test was carried out following the manufacturer's protocol. The initial measurement was taken as the baseline, and no additional compounds were added during this step. Then the OCR was measured with sequential injections of 1.5 µM oligomycin, 2.0 µM carbonyl cyanide 4-(trifluoromethoxy) phenylhydrazone (FCCP, Sigma #C2920), and 0.5 µM RAA. We carried out three repetitions of measurements to obtain average values for each stage (baseline, oligomycin, FCCP, RAA). Each measurement involved three steps: mixing for 3 minutes, waiting for 0 minutes, and measuring for 3 minutes. The mitochondrial respiration was analyzed using Agilent Seahorse Wave Pro software and Mito Stress Test Report Generator.

**Statistical analysis**

The data were expressed as the mean ± standard error of the mean (SEM) and analyzed using Prism 9 (GraphPad Software, Boston, MA). The unpaired Student's $t$-test was used to compare two groups, while a one-way analysis of variance (ANOVA) was used for comparing more than two groups.

## Metabolic profile of murine corneal biopsy

To study the metabolic profile of murine cornea, corneal biopsies in 1.5-mm diameter were used to evaluate the real-time ATP production with the epithelium side up by a Seahorse XFe96 pro Analyzer. Figure 4.1A-B showed that in the fresh isolated adult murine corneal biopsy, 84.3 ± 1.4% of total ATP was produced by oxidative phosphorylation, while only 15.7 ± 1.4% was from glycolysis. This result suggested that mitochondrial metabolism plays a predominant role in the cornea.

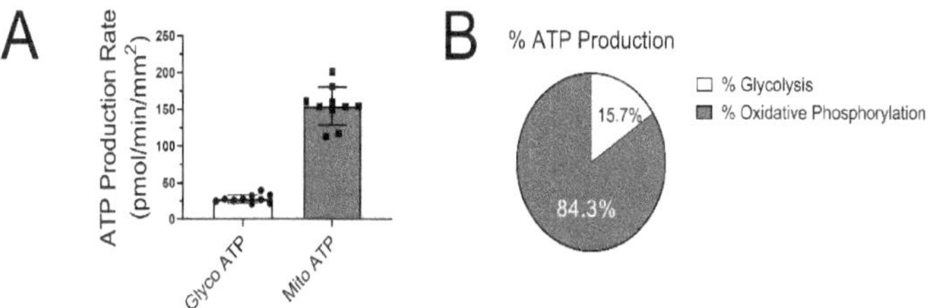


**Figure 4.1 Metabolic profile of murine corneal biopsy.**
(A) ATP production from glycolysis (Glyco) and mitochondria (Mito) were measured in 1.5-mm diameter corneal punches with the epithelium side up from 8-week-old male C57BL/6J mice (n = 10) using real-time ATP rate assay. Values are expressed as mean ± SEM. (B) The average percentages of ATP production from glycolysis and oxidative phosphorylation in murine corneal biopsy (n = 10).

## Different euthanasia methods did not affect OCR in the murine cornea

Given the possibility that the different methods of euthanasia may impact on mitochondrial activity, it is important to evaluate if euthanasia methods can influence OCR in the murine cornea. We performed the Mitochondrial stress assay on corneal biopsy punches in 1.5-mm diameter from male C57BL/6J mice (8-week-old) euthanized either by carbon dioxide asphyxiation or overdosed anesthetic drugs. The results showed no significant difference in basal respiration, maximal respiration, and spare respiration capacities in corneal biopsies between the two euthanasia methods (Fig. 4.2A-D), suggesting that both euthanasia methods are suitable for this assay.

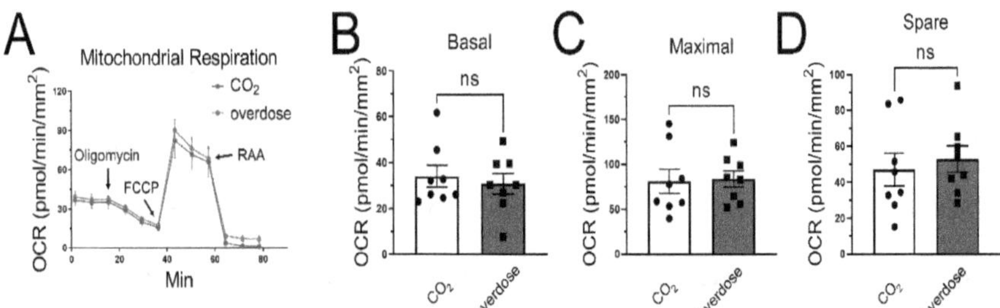

**Figure 4.2 The impact of different euthanasia methods on mouse corneal oxygen consumption.**
(A) Mitochondrial stress test in the corneal biopsies from male C57BL/6J mice euthanized by carbon dioxide asphyxiation (CO2) and an overdose of the anesthetic drug (overdose). (B-D) Statistic analysis graphs of basal, maximal, and spare mitochondrial respiration capacities. Values are expressed as mean ± SEM, n = 8. ns, non-significant.

### Relationship between corneal punch size and OCR values

Agilent recommends OCR values between 20–200 pmol/min prior to normalization as reliable measurements (187). To optimize punch size to yield the optimal OCR value, we performed a mitochondrial stress assay on corneal biopsies with the size of 1.0-mm (size 1.0-mm) and 1.5-mm (size 1.5-mm) in diameter. Corneas were dissected from 8-week-old male C57BL/6J mice euthanized by carbon dioxide asphyxiation. Size 1.0-mm yielded lower OCR recording curves which were below the recommended range, and some biopsies showed poor/flat OCR curves (Fig. 4.3A). The OCR value from size 1.5-mm started from 20 pmol/min and reached the peak of 140 pmol/min after FFCP injection, which was in the optimal range as recommended (Fig. 4.3A-B). After normalization by the biopsy area, size 1.0-mm showed significantly lower maximal and spare respiration capacity and higher variabilities relative to size 1.5-mm. However, there was no significant difference in basal respiration between size 1.0-mm and size 1.5-mm after normalization by the area (Fig. 4.3C-F). Some size 1.0-mm biopsies showed negative values on maximal respiration and spare respiration capacity, suggesting possible mechanical damage and decreased viable cells in tissue biopsies, causing variability for analysis. Thus, mouse corneal biopsy punches in 1.5-mm diameter were more appropriate for mitochondrial activity assays than those in 1.0-mm diameter.

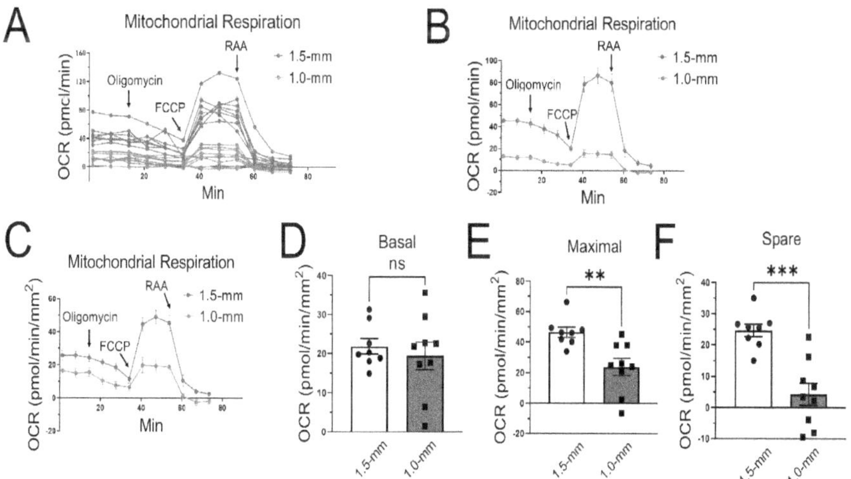

**Figure 4.3 The impact of punch sizes on mouse corneal oxygen consumption.**
(A) Plot showing OCR curve of individual corneal punches in 1.0-mm (red) and 1.5-mm (blue) diameter. (B-C) Mitochondrial stress test using corneal punches of 1.0-mm diameter (n = 10) and 1.5-mm diameter (n = 8) prior to normalization(B) and after normalization by the area of punches (C). (D-F) OCR values in the corneal punches of 1.0-mm diameter (n = 10) and 1.5-mm diameter (n = 8) after normalization by the area of punches. Values are expressed as mean ± SEM. ns, non-significant. ** P < 0.01; *** P < 0.001.

## Relationship between biopsy orientation and corneal OCR values

To assess whether the orientation of corneal biopsies results in different OCR values, we performed a mitochondrial stress assay on corneal biopsies (size 1.5-mm) with either the epithelium or endothelium side upward (facing the cartridge sensor). The results demonstrated no significant difference in the basal, maximal, and spare OCR values between the wells with the epithelial layer facing upward and those with the endothelium side up (Fig. 4.4A-D).

**Relationship between biopsy punch location and corneal OCR values**

Considering that corneal epithelial cells in the center are more mature than those in the periphery, it is intriguing to elucidate the impact of corneal biopsy location on OCR values. We used size 1.5-mm punches from the central and peripheral areas (without limbus) of the cornea from 8-week-old male C57BL/6J mice euthanized by carbon dioxide asphyxiation. The results (Fig. 4.4E-H) showed no significant difference in mitochondrial activity between the punches from the corneal central and peripheral (without limbus) areas.

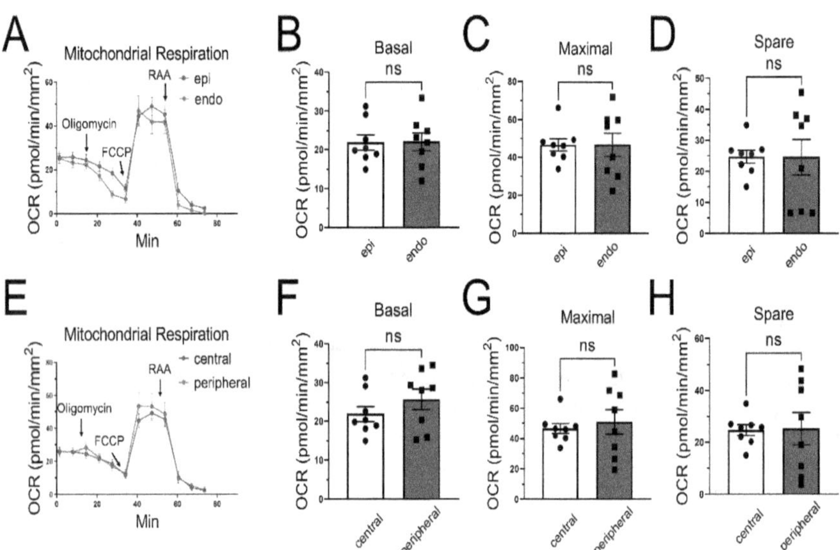

**Figure 4.4 The impact of biopsy orientation and biopsy locations on mouse corneal oxygen consumption.**
(A-D) The OCR values in the murine corneal biopsy with the epithelial layer (epi) and endothelium (endo) facing upward (n = 8). (E-H) The mitochondrial OCR in the punches from the central or peripheral areas of the corneas. Values are expressed as mean ± SEM, n = 8. ns, non-significant.

**The impact of sex, strain, and age of mice on corneal OCR values**

To investigate if there is sexual dimorphism in mitochondrial metabolism, we tested the real-time mitochondrial respiration using the size 1.5-mm cornea punches with the epithelium side up from 8-week-old C57BL/6J mice. Although female corneas showed a trend of higher oxygen consumption than males, there was no significant difference in OCR levels between genders using an unpaired Student's *t*-test (Fig. 4.5A-D).

To study the mouse strain difference in corneal mitochondrial metabolism between pigmented C57BL/6J and albino BALB/cJ mice, we compared the real-time mitochondrial respiration using central corneal punches (size 1.5-mm) with the epithelium side up from 8-week-old male mice. Figure 4.5E-H showed no statistically significant difference in OCR levels between C57BL/6J and BALB/cJ mice.

To compare the corneal mitochondria function in different ages, we measured the OCR values in central corneal biopsies (size 1.5-mm) with the epithelial side up from 4-, 8-, and 32-week-old male C57BL/6J mice. The results showed no significant differences in corneal OCR levels among these ages (Fig. 4.5I-L).

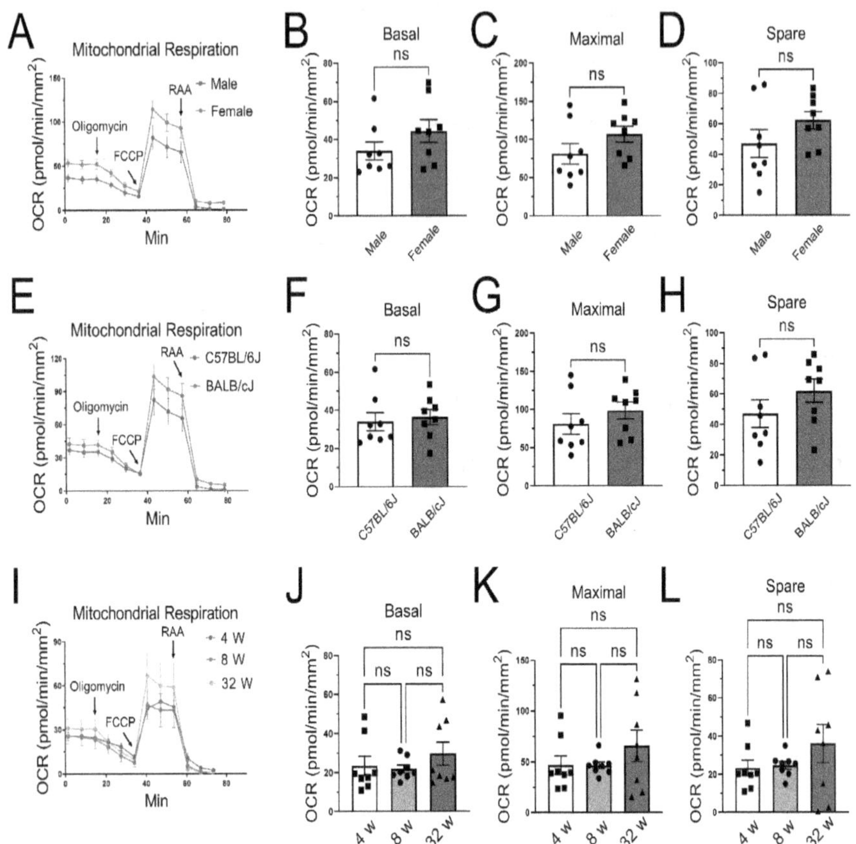


**Figure 4.5 The impacts of sex, strain, and age on murine corneal OCR values.**
(A-D) Mitochondrial stress test in the corneal punches from male and female C57BL/6J mice (n = 8). (E-H) The OCR levels in the cornea punches from C57BL/6J and BALB/cJ mice (n = 8). (I-L) Mitochondrial stress test in the corneas from 4-, 8- and 32-week-old male mice (n = 8). Values are expressed as mean ± SEM. ns, non-significant.

## Mitochondrial respiration in wounded corneas

To track mitochondrial activity in the corneal wound healing process, we generated corneal wounds in 8-week-old male C57BL/6J mice by corneal epithelial debridement. On the day of corneal abrasion (day 0), diminished OCR was detected in the corneal biopsies compared with the unwounded corneas, likely due to the loss of epithelial cells (Fig. 4.6A-D). At day 3 after corneal abrasion, there was a partial recovery of the OCR values, suggesting that mitochondrial activity was affected by the wound-healing process in the cornea.

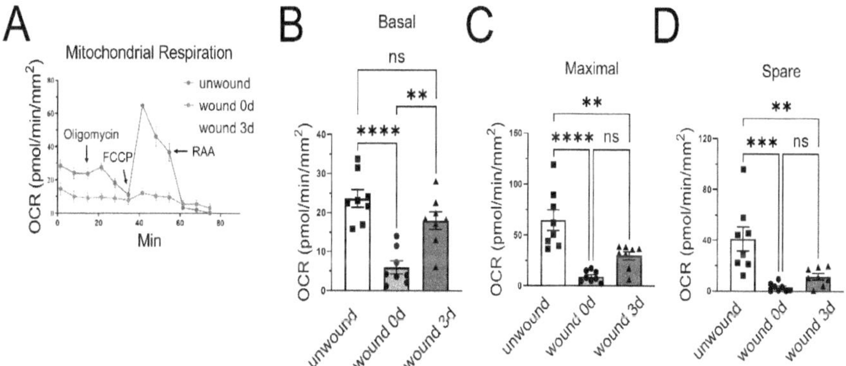


**Figure 4.6 Mitochondrial respiration measurement in wounded corneas.**
(A-D) Mitochondrial stress test in the unwounded cornea and corneas at 0 d and 3 d after wound (n = 8). Values are expressed as mean ± SEM. ns, non-significant; ** P < 0.01; *** P < 0.001; **** P < 0.0001.

## DISCUSSION

Glycolysis and mitochondrial oxidative phosphorylation are two major sources of ATP production in tissues/cells. Therefore, to assess corneal mitochondrial function more precisely, it is necessary to measure mitochondrial function in live cornea biopsies. In this study, we developed and characterized a method to analyze the metabolic profile and mitochondrial function in live murine corneal biopsy using a Seahorse extracellular flux analyzer. Although previous reports have demonstrated the use of Seahorse assay in retinal biopsies (188; 189; 190), to our knowledge, there has been no prior report using corneal biopsies for mitochondrial analysis. Using this novel method, we found that in the live cornea, mitochondrial oxidative phosphorylation is the predominant source of ATP production. This observation emphasized the importance of mitochondrial functional study in the cornea using live murine corneal biopsies. This technique could also assess mitochondrial function in human and other animal corneas. However, the optimal conditions (such as biopsy size and compound concentration) for applying this method to other species need further investigation.

Several studies showed that metabolic profiles of different organs/tissues might be influenced by different anesthesia or euthanasia methods (191; 192). In the present study, for the first time, we compared corneal mitochondrial activity following two commonly used euthanasia methods, an overdose of ketamine/xylazine and carbon dioxide asphyxiation. Our data suggested that no significant differences were detected in corneal OCR values between these two euthanasia methods, indicating that both euthanasia methods can be used for this assay.

The thickness of the murine cornea is ideal to fit within the 0.25 mm deep circular flat detent in each well of the Seahorse 96-well spheroid microplate (193). The detents allowed us to confine the corneal biopsy punches in the center of each well during the assay without using the tissue/cell adhesive such as Cell-Tak. In studies of retina, 1.0-mm in-diameter punches were widely used for real-time measurement of OCR (188; 189; 190). However, we observed a suppressed maximal and spare OCR in corneal punches with a 1.0-mm diameter, falling below the recommended range. In contrast, biopsies of 1.5-mm in diameter generated higher and more reproducible OCR readings within the range recommended by the manufacturer. After normalization by punch area, OCR values from size 1.0-mm biopsies were still lower than those from size 1.5-mm biopsies. Further, some size 1.0-mm punches generated negative OCR values, which resulted in higher variability in OCR relative to size 1.5-mm. Preparation of a size 1.0-mm biopsy may cause tears in the corneal tissue during the punch operation, which could introduce tissue damage that causes loss of mitochondrial activity. Moreover, corneal punches in a 1.0-mm diameter may be curling and result in tissue movement during the assay, which interferes with OCR readings. Therefore, we recommend a 1.5-mm diameter biopsy for the mouse corneal OCR evaluation.

Strain differences in metabolism have been reported in other tissues (194; 195; 196; 197). For example, BALB/cJ mice are known to have a substantially faster visual cycle, suggesting a higher metabolic rate in the retina and RPE relative to C57BL/6J mice (198). In addition, C57BL/6J mice have more severe ischemia-induced retinal neovascularization than BALB/cJ mice (199). Therefore, the genetic background of mice, especially in genetically modified mice, should be carefully considered. Here, we compared corneal mitochondrial activities in these two mouse strains. Unlike the retina, however, we found that BALB/cJ and C57BL/6J mice have similar OCR in corneal biopsies, suggesting no major strain difference in corneal mitochondrial activities, at least between the 2 examined mouse strains.

Age and sex are two other important factors that affect metabolism (200; 201). For example, the mitochondrial volume and density, mitochondrial DNA copy number, and mitochondrial protein levels decrease with aging in the rodent liver (202; 203). Female mice show more mitochondrial biogenesis in the heart and brain than males (204). Female rats express a higher mitochondrial capacity than males in the liver and brown adipose tissue (205; 206). Therefore, we assessed the possible impacts of sex and age on corneal mitochondrial activities. Although a trend of higher OCR was observed in female mice, our results demonstrated no statistically significant difference between males and females in OCR value, at least under physiological conditions. Similarly, we did not observe significant difference among mice at ages 4, 8, and 32 weeks under physiological conditions. However, whether there is a gender or age difference under disease or stress conditions remains to be studied.

Corneal diseases such as diabetic keratopathy, Fuchs' endothelial corneal dystrophy (FECD), and keratoconus have been reported to be associated with disrupted metabolic processes, mitochondrial dysfunction, and decreased ATP production (207; 208; 209). Mitochondrial stress assays can provide valuable insight into the underlying pathophysiology of these conditions. Several mouse models have been developed to study corneal diseases, such as those with mutations in the transcription factor 4 (*TCF4*) gene for FECD and mutations in the visual system homeobox 1 (*VSX1*) gene for keratoconus (210; 211). By measuring corneal OCR in these mouse models, we may be able to better understand the mitochondrial dysfunction underlying these diseases, potentially leading to new therapeutic targets for the treatment of these conditions.

Although assessing mitochondrial function in the live corneal tissue has advantages over the measurement using cultured cells, this method has its limitations as well. The whole corneal biopsy punch may not be amenable to identifying which layers/cell types have altered mitochondrial respiration. To measure the metabolic activities in the isolated corneal stroma, we scratched off the epithelial layer and/or endothelial layer for Seahorse analysis. At day 0 of corneal abrasion, the bare stroma showed a very low OCR value (Fig. 4.6). This could be ascribed to the operation of the corneal tissue, which may induce mechanical damage to other layers, altering the mitochondrial respiration measurement. It may also reflect that the stroma contains very low cell density, and stromal cells primarily use glycolysis to generate ATP (212). The variability of OCR levels on isolated corneal layers was relatively large, and a careful and consistent procedure for punching the cornea is needed.

Corneal epithelium wound by debridement is a commonly used model for corneal wound healing. Our study using corneal biopsy punches taken from different timepoint after corneal epithelial debridement revealed that trauma/wound healing alters mitochondrial respiration in the cornea. Specifically, corneal epithelial wound decreased OCR values in the corneal biopsies compared to unwounded corneas. Recovery of the OCR values was associated with corneal wound healing, which suggested that mitochondrial function is required for the maintenance of physiopathology activity in the cornea. Low OCR values at day 0 of the wound are likely due to the loss of epithelial cells. Previous studies showed the corneal wounds were completely healed, which was confirmed by sodium fluorescein staining, in this model at day 3 (145; 213; 214; 215; 216; 217). Surprisingly, the OCR value on day 3 was still significantly lower than the unwounded cornea. This lower OCR may be explained by the fact that the cell number may not be completely recovered to the unwounded level at day 3. It is also possible that proliferating epithelial cells at the wounded area may use glycolysis rather than mitochondrial oxidative phosphorylation. Future studies will be required to measure glycolysis in the wounded area and to elucidate the cause of the changes in mitochondrial functions in the newly healed cornea. Additionally, some chemicals, proteins, and drugs have been discovered to have therapeutic benefits in the context of corneal wound healing and fibrosis (110; 128; 218; 219; 220). It is of great interest to investigate whether these therapeutic effects are associated with corneal mitochondrial function and ATP production.

To obtain reproducible OCR measurements, we normalized the OCR values by the punch area and kept the biopsy punch size consistent. This is a well-accepted method to minimize the need for secondary normalization. However, in certain situations, such as corneal epithelial wounds, an external normalization factor may be necessary based on cell counts, total protein concentration, or genomic DNA copy numbers.

In summary, we optimized a method for examining mitochondrial respiration in live murine cornea. The findings provided important information for researchers seeking to study the mitochondrial function of the cornea.

## CHAPTER V

## DISCUSSION AND SUMMARY

### DISCUSSION

In people with diabetes, the healing process of corneal wounds can be slower. Delayed corneal epithelial wound healing may lead to sight-threatening complications, including ocular surface irregularities, microbial keratitis and corneal scarring (93). Increasing evidence suggests that various corneal components (epithelium, stroma, nerves, and endothelium) are affected by diabetes (111; 112). Currently, there is no effective therapeutic strategy for diabetic keratopathy, as the molecular mechanism for the diabetes-induced corneal wound healing deficiency remains elusive.

The Wnt/β-catenin signaling is a complex and highly conserved pathway that plays a crucial role in a wide range of biological processes, including development, cell proliferation, differentiation, and stem cell maintenance (29; 113; 114; 115). Dysregulation of the Wnt signaling pathway has been linked to various diseases, including diabetes, cancer, osteoporosis, and neurodegenerative disorders (221; 222; 223; 224). Wnt signaling dysregulation in diabetes conditions is tissue specific. For example, we found that Wnt signaling is over-activated in the retina from diabetic patients or diabetic animal models (31; 32; 42). Furthermore, aberrant activation of canonical Wnt signaling leads to retinal inflammation and neovascularization (31; 32; 40; 41; 42). However, diabetes suppressed Wnt signaling in the skin and delayed skin wound healing (52). Recently, a study suggested that Wnt signaling may mediate the beneficial effect of insulin on corneal wound healing (61). Despite its importance, the specific role of Wnt/β-catenin signaling in the process of corneal wound repair is not fully understood. The study presented in this dissertation found evidence that kallistatin, an endogenous inhibitor of Wnt signaling, is increased in the corneas of diabetic patients and animal models. Interestingly, even in the absence of diabetes, kallistatin overexpression or administration was found to suppress Wnt signaling and delay corneal wound healing. This suggests that diabetes-induced increases of kallistatin play a significant role in impairing corneal epithelial wound healing through the suppression of Wnt/β-catenin signaling. Further experiments with Wnt activators and inhibitors showed that canonical Wnt signaling plays a crucial role in corneal wound healing, and that diabetes suppresses Wnt signaling in the cornea, leading to impaired wound healing. These findings provide evidence that in the cornea, where Wnt signaling is required for proper wound healing, kallistatin-mediated inhibition of the Wnt pathway can impair wound healing.

The impaired wound healing in diabetic skin and cornea may be due to the low-level inflammation that is characteristic of diabetes (225). Inflammation can be a double-edged sword, as it is necessary for the initial stages of wound healing, but excessive or prolonged inflammation can delay healing and lead to chronic wounds. The depressed Wnt signaling pathway has been implicated in the impaired wound healing observed in diabetic skin and cornea, which may be linked to chronic low-level inflammation, but it is not clear if kallistatin is the primary mediator of this effect. Overall, the relationship between kallistatin, Wnt signaling, and wound healing in diabetes is complex and multifaceted. While kallistatin may play a role in the impaired wound healing observed in diabetic skin and cornea, further research is needed to fully understand the mechanisms involved and identify potential therapeutic targets.

Peroxisome proliferator-activated receptor alpha (PPARα) is a protein that belongs to the family of nuclear receptors(63). It plays a vital role in the regulation of various metabolic processes such as fatty acid oxidation, glucose homeostasis, and inflammation (63). Our research, as the second part of this dissertation, delves into the role of PPARα signaling and mitochondrial function in the impaired wound healing process in the cornea of individuals with diabetes. By treating STZ-induced diabetic mouse with a PPARα agonist, we were able to alleviate corneal mitochondrial dysfunction and the associated delay in corneal wound healing, which was substantiated by the role of PPARα in the mitochondrial function and wound healing of cornea. However, studying the specific role of PPARα in corneal wound healing using global *PPARα* knockout mice can be challenging due to other physiological processes caused by systemic metabolic changes in *PPARα*[-/-] mice. Global knockout of *PPARα* can cause severe metabolic disturbances and organ dysfunction, which may confound the interpretation of the wound healing results. To gain a more targeted and precise understanding of the role of PPARα in corneal wound healing, we generated tissue-specific conditional *PPARα* knockout mice with deletion of PPARα specifically in corneal epithelium, while preserving its function in other tissues. Conditional knockout of *PPARα* in the corneal epithelium leads to declines in corneal mitochondrial function and impaired wound healing. In contrast, overexpression of *PPARα* in the corneal epithelium showed improvement in mitochondrial function and corneal wound healing. Our findings suggest that mitochondrial dysfunction is a key factor in the reduced wound healing capacity in the diabetic cornea and that PPARα plays a crucial role in regulating this mitochondrial function in the corneal epithelium. These results provide valuable insights into potential therapeutic targets for diabetic keratopathy.

Mitochondrial dysfunction has been identified as a key contributor to the development of diabetic complications. Diabetic patients have been found to exhibit reduced mitochondrial function, which can contribute to the development of various diabetic complications, including diabetic peripheral neuropathy, diabetic nephropathy, diabetic retinopathy, and diabetic cardiomyopathy (135; 136; 137; 159; 160). Mitochondria are known as the powerhouses of the cell, as they generate energy in the form of ATP through oxidative phosphorylation. In diabetes, the impairment of mitochondrial function can lead to decreased ATP production, which can result in insufficient energy supply to cells, including those involved in the process of wound healing. This decrease in ATP production can lead to slower cell migration and proliferation, which are essential processes for wound healing. Furthermore, mitochondria play a critical role in regulating reactive oxygen species (ROS) levels in tissues/cells. ROS are known to have both beneficial and detrimental effects on cells, but in excess, they can cause cellular damage and promote inflammation. In diabetes, impaired mitochondrial function can lead to an increase in ROS production, which can result in oxidative stress, a state where there is an imbalance between ROS production and the body's ability to detoxify them. This oxidative stress can further exacerbate the already compromised wound healing process in the diabetic cornea, as it can contribute to inflammation and cell death. In this dissertation, we discovered that human corneal epithelial cells primarily rely on mitochondrial oxidation for energy production, while corneal stromal fibroblasts primarily utilize glycolysis. Furthermore, we found that mitochondrial function was significantly reduced in the diabetic cornea. The decrease in ATP and increase in ROS due to impaired mitochondrial function can have detrimental effects on corneal wound healing. It can result in delayed or incomplete wound closure, prolonged inflammation, and increased susceptibility to infection. Addressing mitochondrial dysfunction, either through targeting PPARα signaling or other therapeutic strategies, could potentially help alleviate these effects and improve the wound healing process in diabetic individuals.

In order to assess mitochondrial function in a more accurate and *in vivo* like manner, it is important to measure mitochondrial oxygen consumption in live tissues. However, traditional methods of mitochondrial isolation and *in vitro* measurement using cultured cells have limitations such as disruption of cell/organelle structures and alteration of the tissular/cellular micro-environments and cell-to-cell interactions (183). To address these limitations, the third part of this dissertation aimed to develop a more sophisticated and efficient assay for real-time measurement of mitochondrial metabolism in live murine corneal tissue using the Seahorse XFe96 Extracellular Flux Analyzer. This study examined the conditions that could impact the measurement such as the impact of different euthanasia methods, punch sizes, and biopsy locations on the measurement of oxygen consumption rate (OCR) in the cornea. Moreover, the OCR values between different mouse sexes, ages, and strains were also compared to provide a comprehensive evaluation of mitochondrial function in the murine cornea. These results will provide a valuable tool for researchers to study the impact of various factors on mitochondrial function in the cornea, which can be beneficial in understanding and treating corneal wound healing deficiencies in diabetes.

The relationship between Wnt signaling and mitochondrial function is not well established. Recent evidence suggests that Wnt signaling can interact and regulate mitochondrial function in various ways. Large-scale RNAi screen showed that Wnt3a is a potent activator of mitochondrial biogenesis and oxidative phosphorylation gene expression in C2C12 mouse muscle cell line (226). Similarly, it was reported that Wnt3α promotes mitochondrial biogenesis in adipocytes (227). There was a study that suggested β-catenin knocking down decreased mitochondrial biogenesis in breast cancer cells (228). Our unpublished data also suggested that activation of Wnt signaling promotes mitochondrial function in the cornea. There is limited evidence suggesting that the Wnt signaling and PPARα pathways may interact and regulate each other in some contexts. For example, our studies have suggested that PPARα agonist suppressed Wnt3a-induced Wnt signaling in renal cells (130). Activation of Wnt-signaling pathway reverses the suppressive effect of PPARα antagonist in endometrial epithelial cells (229). Wnt signaling can affect PPARα expression and activity, while PPARα can modulate Wnt signaling by altering the expression of Wnt ligands and receptors in certain neurodegenerative diseases (230; 231). Further research is needed to fully understand the relationship between the Wnt pathway and PPARα signaling in the regulation of mitochondrial function and cellular processes in the cornea.

Despite what we found regarding the pathogenesis of diabetic keratopathy, there are many unanswered questions that remain to be addressed. One of the key factors that remains poorly understood is the regulation of kallistatin. Our studies have revealed that diabetes-induced upregulation of kallistatin may contribute to the impaired corneal wound healing through inhibition of the canonical Wnt signaling pathway. However, it is not yet clear what regulates the expression of kallistatin in the cornea as well as the circulation, and whether it could serve as a biomarker for diabetic keratopathy. Furthermore, the potential efficacy of kallistatin inhibition as a cure for diabetic keratopathy is unknown. While kallistatin/Wnt/β-catenin signaling has been shown to play a role in diabetic keratopathy, it is not yet clear if Wnt activators have the direct therapeutic impact on diabetic keratopathy. In addition to the role of kallistatin, the mechanisms behind kallistatin's differential effects on various tissues, such as the cornea and skin compared to the retina and kidney, are also not yet fully understood. It is important to determine why kallistatin has different effects on these tissues. Another aspect that requires further investigation is the role of Wnt/β-catenin signaling in corneal mitochondrial function. The exact relationship between Wnt signaling and corneal mitochondrial function remains unclear and requires further study. Finally, the relationship between Wnt signaling and PPARα in the cornea is also not well understood. Further investigation is needed to determine the relationship or crosstalk between these two signaling pathways in the cornea.

Taken together, we identified for the first time that corneal epithelial cells rely on mitochondria-generated oxidative phosphorylation as a major source of ATP energy. This discovery sheds light on the important role of mitochondria in maintaining corneal health and supports further exploration of the potential link between mitochondrial dysfunction and impaired wound healing in diabetic cornea. This dissertation also highlights that downregulation of Wnt/β-catenin signaling and PPARα level plays a pathogenic role in wound healing deficiency in diabetic cornea. By focusing on Wnt signaling, the PPARα pathway and mitochondrial function, we hope to better understand the mechanisms behind diabetic keratopathy and ultimately develop effective treatments.

# SUMMARY

Despite advances in medical technology, current treatments for diabetic keratopathy remain limited. The lack of effective treatments for diabetic keratopathy is a major concern, as it can cause significant vision impairment and even blindness in severe cases. Despite the prevalence of diabetes, the underlying mechanisms of diabetic keratopathy remain poorly understood, and there is a great need for more research in this area.

The aim of this dissertation is to gain insights into the dysregulation of cornea wound healing in diabetes. The results showed that increased levels of kallistatin, an endogenous inhibitor of Wnt signaling, were found in diabetic corneas from human patients, rats, and mice. The activation of canonical Wnt signaling was suppressed in the wounded cornea of diabetic mice, which corresponded to delayed wound healing. Additionally, transgenic expression of kallistatin suppressed the activation of the corneal Wnt signaling and exacerbated the delay in corneal wound healing. The manipulation of Wnt signaling in the cornea using inhibitors or activators was found to regulate the rate of corneal wound healing. These findings suggest that diabetes-induced overexpression of kallistatin contributes to the delay in corneal wound healing by inhibiting the canonical Wnt signaling pathway, providing a new therapeutic target for the treatment of diabetic keratopathy. Our studies have demonstrated that levels of PPARα in the corneal epithelium are significantly reduced in both diabetic patients and diabetic animal models, and this reduction correlates with impaired mitochondrial function and delayed corneal wound healing. To further investigate the molecular mechanisms underlying this relationship, we used multiple experimental approaches including genetic manipulations, drug treatments, and RNA interference. Our results demonstrated that PPARα deficiency, either through global or epithelium-specific knockout, leads to decreased mitochondrial function and impaired corneal wound healing, while activation of PPARα using a specific agonist ameliorates the mitochondrial dysfunction or epithelium-specific overexpression improves corneal mitochondrial function and wound healing. These findings provide strong evidence that the downregulation of PPARα is a key contributor to the impaired mitochondrial function and delayed wound healing in the diabetic cornea.

In summary, decreased Wnt signaling together with PPARα levels in the cornea may contribute to the pathogenesis of diabetic keratopathy in part. Our studies have important implications for the development of therapeutic strategies for the treatment of diabetic corneal wound healing defects. Further investigations are needed to elucidate the roles of the canonical Wnt pathway and PPARα signaling, as well as their interactions, in corneal wound healing.